New Technologies in Surgical Oncology

Antonio Mussa (Ed.)

New Technologies in Surgical Oncology

Foreword by
Enrico De Antoni

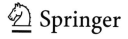 Springer

Editor
Antonio Mussa
Surgical Oncology Unit
S. Giovanni Battista University Hospital
Turin, Italy

ISBN 978-88-470-1474-9   e-ISBN 978-88-470-1475-6

DOI 10.1007/978-88-470-1475-6

Springer Dordrecht Heidelberg London Milan New York

Library of Congress Control Number: 2009936073

Cover design: Simona Colombo, Milan, Italy

Typesetting: Graphostudio, Milan, Italy
Printing and binding: Arti Grafiche Nidasio, Assago (MI), Italy
Printed in Italy

Springer-Verlag Italia S.r.l. – Via Decembrio 28 – I-20137 Milan
Springer is a part of Springer Science+Business Media (www.springer.com)

Foreword

The Italian Society of Surgery has taken the opportunity to offer its members and the medical community at large an update on new technologies in the detection and treatment of neoplastic pathologies. Progress achieved over the last few decades, especially in the field of oncology, has been unstoppable, necessitating an update on the methods used to examine patients and in turn the therapeutic protocols used in their treatment. Despite concerns over the enormous increase in the cost of healthcare, there is an irresistible drive by physicians and medical institutions to acquire state-of-the-art systems and to apply the most recently developed methods.

The Italian Society of Surgery has entrusted the subject of the Bi-annual, 2009 Report to Antonio Mussa, an internationally famous oncologist and surgeon, Director of the Oncology Department of the "Molinette" Hospital of Torino, and President of the Oncology Commission of Piemonte. Prof. Mussa has addressed many of the innovative scientific advancements in the 350 articles he has published to date and in the many congresses and meetings he has organized. His experience covers a wide range of medical specialties, from breast receptors to radio-immuno-guided surgery of various organs. His organizational skills have led to the creation of the Piemonte Oncological Network, the first and only such structure in Italy.

This volume is a particularly interesting scientific publication, of great significance to today's clinical practice. As President of the Italian Society of Surgery, it is with great pride that I present this work. I sincerely recommend it to surgeons and oncologists as an excellent guide, one that covers all the therapeutic options in the treatment of neoplasms. The book's detailed suggestions and explanations will facilitate the choice of the best treatment for patients, in terms of both cure and preservation of function.

Rome, October 2009

Enrico De Antoni
President
Italian Society of Surgery

v

Preface

I would like to thank the President and Board of Trustees of the Italian Society of Surgery for the opportunity to realize this important task, as well as all those who cooperated in the achievement of this project, particularly Professor Sergio Sandrucci, for his invaluable cooperation and support.

Oncological surgery consists of a moment in the diagnostic-therapeutic course of the patient. The outstanding progress that has taken place in the field of oncology in the last two decades has benefited from the development of new surgical techniques, which have allowed highly specialized oncological surgery and a surgical approach more thoroughly integrated within the context of multidisciplinary oncological treatment. Indeed, it is no longer acceptable that a surgeon care for an oncology patient without having broad therapeutic and diagnostic knowledge of the opportunities offered by other fields of medicine.

After many years of experience in general medicine, and after 20 years as Rector of the Institute of Oncological Specialization, I was eager to leave my own personal mark in the evolution of oncological surgery.

At the Oncological Institute, together with my colleagues, partners, and students, I have developed two post-graduate University Masters programs, one dealing with Palliative Care and the other with Oncological Surgery, which offer much more than the standard surgical knowledge. Undoubtedly, the aim of this collection of techniques, currently the most modern in this field, is to diffuse different types of knowledge and skills to other surgeons, in order to not only improve the lifespan of the oncological patient but also to preserve its quality.

Turin, October 2009

Antonio Mussa
Surgical Oncology Unit
S. Giovanni Battista University Hospital
Turin

Contents

List of Contributors

Alberto Arezzo
Centre of Mini-Invasive Surgery
S. Giovanni Battista University Hospital
Turin, Italy

Paolo Bogetti
Plastic Surgery Unit
S. Giovanni Battista University Hospital
Turin, Italy

Enrico Brignardello
Oncological Endocrinology Service
S. Giovanni Battista University Hospital
Turin, Italy

Stefano Bruschi
Plastic Surgery Unit
S. Giovanni Battista University Hospital
Turin, Italy

Riccardo Bussone
Breast surgery unit
S. Giovanni Battista University Hospital
Turin, Italy

Giulia Carbonaro
Liver Translantation Unit - General
Surgery 8
S. Giovanni Battista University Hospital
Turin, Italy

Piero Celoria
Surgical Oncology Unit
S. Giovanni Battista University Hospital
Turin, Italy

Alessandro Comandone
Department of Medical Oncology
Gradenigo Hospital
Turin, Italy

Marisa Deandrea
Oncological Endocrine Surgery Service
S. Giovanni Battista University Hospital
Turin, Italy

Claudio De Angelis
Echoendoscopy Service and
GEP Neuroendocrine Tumors Center
Department of GastroHepatology
S. Giovanni Battista University Hospital
Turin, Italy

Riccardo Ferracini
Orthopedics and Traumatology Unit
S. Giovanni Battista University Hospital
Turin, Italy

Alessandra Galetto
Clinical Oncology
Ospedale della Carità
Novara, Italy

Matteo Goss
Surgical Oncology Unit
S. Giovanni Battista University Hospital
Turin, Italy

Tommaso Lubrano
Surgical Oncology Unit
S. Giovanni Battista University Hospital
Turin, Italy

Patrizia Marsanic
Surgical Oncology Unit
S. Giovanni Battista University Hospital
Turin, Italy

Lina Matera
Clinical Immunology
S. Giovanni Battista University Hospital
Turin, Italy

Alberto Mobiglia
Surgical Oncology Unit
S. Giovanni Battista University Hospital
Turin, Italy

Mario Morino
Centre of Mini-Invasive Surgery
S. Giovanni Battista University Hospital
Turin, Italy

Rosa Moscato
Surgical Oncology Unit
S. Giovanni Battista University Hospital
Turin, Italy

Antonio Mussa
Surgical Oncology Unit
S. Giovanni Battista University Hospital
Turin, Italy

Baudolino Mussa
Surgical Oncology Unit
S. Giovanni Battista University Hospital
Turin, Italy

Alberto Oliaro
Thoracic Surgery
S. Giovanni Battista University Hospital
Turin, Italy

Pietro Panier Suffat
Surgical Oncology Unit
S. Giovanni Battista University Hospital
Turin, Italy

Patrizia Racca
Medical Oncology - C.U.R.O.
S. Giovanni Battista University Hospital
Turin, Italy

Monica Rampino
Oncologic Radiotherapy Unit
S. Giovanni Battista University Hospital
Turin, Italy

Alessia Reali
Oncologic Radiotherapy Unit
S. Giovanni Battista University Hospital
Turin, Italy

Fabrizio Rebecchi
Centre of Mini-Invasive Surgery
Turin, Italy
S. Giovanni Battista University Hospital
Turin, Italy

Lorenzo Repetto
Urology Unit III
S. Giovanni Battista University Hospital
Turin, Italy

Alessandro Repici
Digestive Endoscopy Unit
IRCCS Istituto Clinico Humanitas
Milan, Italy

Umberto Ricardi
Oncologic Radiotherapy Unit
S. Giovanni Battista University Hospital
Turin, Italy

Dorico Righi
Interventional Radiology Unit
S. Giovanni Battista University Hospital
Turin, Italy

Carlo Riccardo Rossi
Sarcoma and Melanoma Unit
Clinica Chirurgica II
University of Padua
Padua, Italy

Enrico Ruffini
Thoracic Surgery
S. Giovanni Battista University Hospital
Turin, Italy

Mauro Salizzoni
Liver Translantation Unit - General
Surgery 8
S. Giovanni Battista University Hospital
Turin, Italy

Sergio Sandrucci
Surgical Oncology Unit
S. Giovanni Battista University Hospital
Turin, Italy

Rosella Spadi
Medical Oncology - C.U.R.O.
S. Giovanni Battista University Hospital
Turin, Italy

Flavio Trombetta
Surgical Oncology Unit
S. Giovanni Battista University Hospital
Turin, Italy

Andrea Veltri
Institute of Radiology
S. Luigi Hospital
University of Turin
Turin, Italy

The Evolution of Surgical Oncology

1

A. Mussa, A. Mobiglia

Providing a description of the history of surgery, which is considered the main therapeutic option for a disease once absolutely incurable, is extremely complex. Cancer is the disease which perhaps more than any other summarises man's past and present fears in the face of his own vulnerability – as claimed and described by Cosmacini and Sironi [1] in their book *"Il male del secolo"* ("The disease of the century") which accurately portrays the history of tumor disease.

From the time when the causal suspicion connected with the "black bile disorder" (also known as "choleric upset") was introduced in *De naturalibus facultatibus* by the physician Claudio Galeno (129–200 A.D.), up until the identification of oncogenes at the origin of many neoplastic forms, evolution in the past has entailed a radical revision of etiopathogenetic mechanisms, as well as therapeutic results. The latter, thanks to the development and integration of a number of practices, have changed appreciably both in terms of survival and recovery of the patient to social life. Nonetheless, the inability to totally control the disease still persists, except in the initial phase and with drastically ablative methods, where still today surgery is the most frequently applied option.

In only one hundred years, a mere blink of the eye since the appearance on Earth of Homo sapiens, the whole of medicine gathered the fruits of the scientific fervor sown by the Renaissance and the Enlightenment. At the dawn of the nineteenth century, defined "the century of surgery", it reached its epitome thanks to two discoveries: anesthetics and antiseptics [2].

Prior to 1846, the year the first operation under ether anesthetic was carried out at the Massachusetts General Hospital, it was not at all strange for the surgeon dressed in a frock coat and with bare hands to operate on patients who were awake, horror-stricken and immobilised by the surgeon's assistants. Indeed coldness and temperament were appreciated in those who operated on the sick without anesthesia.

A. Mussa (✉)
Surgical Oncology Unit, S. Giovanni Battista University Hospital, Turin, Italy

New Technologies in Surgical Oncology. Antonio Mussa (Ed.)
© Springer-Verlag Italia 2010

1

These were the same requisites asked of those wanting to practise surgery indicated by Celso some 1,500 years earlier as indispensable character traits for the profession.

Important intuitions concerning infection were made by Semmelweis, Lister and Pasteur. Infective agents therefore began to find their nosological setting only a few years later following Robert Koch's discoveries and thanks to the importance demonstrated by microorganisms, made possible by the use of the microscope (moreover invented two centuries earlier). Antiseptic treatment extended rapidly from wounds to surgical instruments, then to the rooms and furnishing used, to clothes and the surgeon's hands, and contributed in a decisive way to limiting the till-then devastating damage of infectious diseases.

From antiseptics the next step was to seek asepsis, with operations being performed in closed environments exclusively dedicated to this activity: the first operating theatres were thus born. The surgeon wore more suitable clothes for this dedicated work: in a few years the use of the white coat spread, followed by hair covering (with Neuber), gloves (with Halsted) and finally masks (with von Mikulicz).

Anesthesia and antiseptics meant that in a few decades the surgeon could tackle increasingly difficult and longer operations. Between the end of the nineteenth and the early twentieth centuries many techniques were invented that were valid enough to still be used today: Billroth honed complex gastric surgical procedures, Kocher dealt with thyroid surgery, and Halsted proposed radical mastectomy extending to the lymphatic stations for breast cancer treatment. However, opening the abdominal or thoracic cavity and tackling the skull still proved risky due to the chance of provoking infections not easy to control, and it was only the discovery made by Sir Alexander Fleming of penicillin which provided the surgeon with an efficacious weapon to combat them.

With the advent of epidemiological studies, research on cancerogenous agents, innovations in diagnostic techniques and radiotherapy, oncology in the early 1900s began to be configured as a multidisciplinary investigational science.

At a conference on tumor immunology in 1908, Paul Ehrlich postulated that malignant cells could frequently form during the course of life and that antigenic structures were found on their plasmalemma against which the host produced an antibody response which in most cases was sufficient to eliminate the neoplastic elements. This was the first insight into the importance of the immune system in controlling neoplastic disease.

On the other hand, it began to be conjectured at the same time that cancer derived from "genetic errors" (in 1914, by studying the eggs of sea urchins, the German zoologist Theodor Boveri postulated that cancer was due to chromosome abnormalities).

From the beginning of the century up to the Second World War there were basically two weapons used against cancer: surgery and radiotherapy. However, some discoveries made in the 1940s showed that cancer was not invulnerable to drugs: this marked the dawn of chemotherapy.

In the meantime diagnostic techniques improved and, against the risk of tumors and metastases, prevention and early diagnosis were recommended. An article had already appeared on this subject in 1913 in the American women's magazine 'Ladies' Home Journal', which described tumor symptoms and transferred the risk of mortality from the ruthlessness of the disease to its late surgical treatment. To all effects this was the first publicity campaign for prevention!

In 1946 George Papanicolaou perfected the first method for early diagnosis – the Pap-test for cancer of the uterine cervix. At the time cervical cancer was the most serious and common tumor among women, and the test consequently determined the drastic drop in mortality of this disease.

Farber demonstrated the efficacy of a drug (aminopterine) against leukaemia in children, and, during the same period, Goodman and Gilman together with a thoracic surgeon, Gustav Linskog, administered a mustard gas derivative, mustine, to a patient suffering from non-Hodgkin lymphoma, which led to the drastic reduction of the tumor. They were therefore the first clinical researchers to witness the efficacy of a drug in attempting to halt neoplastic growth, at least temporarily. This took place in 1946–1947.

Important studies were also carried out by C. Huggins, who discovered the therapeutic efficacy of estrogens in breast carcinoma (1940), and orchiectomy in prostate carcinoma (1941), thus introducing the concept of "hormonal control" of tumor development.

Almost simultaneously the first large scientific work of an epidemiological and investigational nature was published in the United States on the correlation between smoking and lung cancer. The attempt to identify all the chemical substances which could cause cancer coincided with the growing awareness on the part of the public of environmental problems: talk thus began of a possible link between the increased rate of cancer and pollution.

The ferment of those years led D.A. Karnofsky to seek to organise tumor treatment in a systematic form: in 1949, in his attempt to make single case studies homogeneous and comparable, he formulated the "validity status" of the tumor patient (subsequently, in 1961, he also dictated the criteria for objective evaluation of the response to anti-proliferative drugs).

It was at Cambridge in 1953 that James Dewey Watson and Francis Harry Compton Crick discovered the DNA double helix structure (for which they received the Nobel Prize in Medicine in 1962), thus laying the cornerstone of the modern era of oncology.

To return to the strictly surgical sphere, the outcome of an operation, apart from the technique adopted, remains largely connected with the skill of the operator. But the human factor, among others, poses a practical and ethical problem. In effect it creates categories of merit based on often debatable judgements which engender confusion and doubt in patients towards the surgeon, whom in most cases they have not had the chance to choose and to whom they are entrusting their life. It is therefore not surprising that there have always been attempts to see this aspect in its true light, trying to limit the influence of individual capacities on the outcome of the operation by adopting protocols and codified procedures, preferably mechanical and therefore automatic. It is even less surprising that this reasoning was fundamental for the birth, in Soviet Moscow of the 1950s, of a "Scientific Research Institute of Experimental Surgical Apparatus and Instruments" where work began to study and make instruments for automatic suture that could be used by all surgeons, even in the farthest hospital of that immense territory so as to ensure standard treatment for an adequate, homogeneous level of care.

In actual fact the need to create automatic suture mechanisms arose much earlier. The strange, remarkable method thought up by Abulcasis in the tenth century should be recalled, whereby for intestinal suture the jaws of a particular type of ant decapitated after it had bitten into tissue were used; or again that of J.B. Murphy who invented a metallic button for intestinal suture in 1892, which would be taken up again almost a century later in Valtrac's invention, a biodegradable ring used for the same purpose.

However, the mechanical suture method intended as a process capable of automatically placing stitches was born at the beginning of the twentieth century. The fist apparatus, perfected in Budapest by Humer Hultl and presented at the Second Congress of the Hungarian Society for Surgery in 1908, deserves a mention. Used in gastric resection, it was able to apply four rows of metallic stitches which, by hermetically fixing the anterior part of the stomach to the posterior part, enabled removal of a portion with no bleeding or spreading of its contents.

A surgeon with expertise in tumor disease could therefore apply the so-called "no touch" techniques in an almost flawless way, with the help of excluding mechanical staplers – the so-called "cut and sew".

However, research also progressed in terms of the patient's quality of life. In 1973 the first clinical trial was started on quadrantectomy for breast cancer, a new surgical technique developed by Umberto Veronesi. It was the first introduction to a conservative operation, the removal of only the diseased part of the breast, with the purpose of reducing patient mutilation. The trial ended successfully in 1981 but only in 2002 was the technique given full recognition by the international scientific community.

From 1982 to 1985, new means for diagnosing tumors were perfected thanks to the progress of information technology. Diagnostic Imaging, for example, has since been used to increase the ability to visualize the details of organs and tissue: from that moment on it became possible to "see" the tumor – even in its initial phases or in parts of the body not accessible to physical examination.

Increasingly effective, more selective and ever less invasive pharmacological therapies were sought: the concept of "therapeutic targets" was born. Proteins and "wrong" genes giving origin to diseases could be hit by made-to-measure drugs able to distinguish between healthy and diseased tissue.

In 1992 Ira Pastan bound a monoclonal antibody able to distinguish healthy cells from tumor cells to a toxin. The result was a sort of guided "bullet" which destroyed diseased tissue while sparing the healthy tissue surrounding it.

By the end of the 1990s the link between genes and cancer had been established. It was now apparent that the disease arises when a critical number of "genetic errors" accumulate in the DNA. This can be confirmed in studies on familiarity, or when there is the co-presence of more than one form of cancer in the same subject. We began to speak of "genic therapy", whereby the "broken" genes could be substituted with ones that functioned.

The Human Genome Project intended to complete the genome inventory, namely the reading of the complete sequence of nitrogen bases composing our genetic code,

and thanks to the extraordinary progress of information technology this was completed in 2000. The gene inventory had become a reality, with researchers laying the
foundations for a great scientific revolution: the post-genomic revolution.

Clinical trials began to deal with a new class of drugs, whose objective was not
so much to kill the tumor cell, but to repair or deactivate it. In more recent years
research has shifted from observation of the gene to its protein (proteomics), which
is actually the molecule which carries out the genetic programme, and then to relations between proteins and metabolic systems of the body (metabolomics). It was
thus understood that the tumor alters the entire surrounding environment to its favor,
exploiting almost all the body's systems (e.g. neoangiogenesis).

Today's surgeon is certainly more eclectic than in the past and needs to have a
wider vision of tumor disease and its problems in order to tackle its treatment with
both traditional and more innovative procedures. These include mini-invasive techniques, endoscopy, laparoscopy (which has taken huge steps both in application criteria and oncological radicality), and robotics, with the achievement of tele-guided
surgery and multidisciplinary integration with imaging diagnostic options directly
usable in the operative field, and performance enhancement of some procedures in
day-surgery as well.

Consequently, at the beginning of the new millennium, the figure is increasingly
emerging of a surgeon specialized in treating tumors, who is fully up to date in diagnostic practice and aware of the non-surgical therapeutic options, and who is an
expert in integrated therapeutic programmes with a multidisciplinary approach.

The oncological surgeon is no longer seen merely as a technical craftsman, but
rather as a faithful presence at the different moments of prevention, diagnosis, treatment and palliation of tumor disease, and shall remain so at least until the recent and
future scientific acquisitions manage to substitute tumor "removal" with absolutely
selective and less invasive methods.

References

1. Cosmacini G, Sironi VA (2002) Il male del secolo. Per una storia del cancro. (The disease of
    the century. A history of cancer) Editore Laterza, Roma–Bari
2. Cosmacini G (2003) La vita nelle mani. Storia della chirurgia. (Life in their hands. The his-
    tory of surgery). Editori Laterza, Roma–Bari

Minimally Invasive Techniques in Surgical Oncology

2

M. Morino, A. Arezzo, E. Ruffini, A. Oliaro

Introduction

Minimally invasive surgery for cancer is an emerging concept, now that it has achieved established success in the treatment of several benign diseases. Nevertheless mature data on the safety of these procedures is keenly awaited, as to date they are mostly restricted to the field of colon cancer.

While awaiting these confirmations a new challenge is already knocking on the door [1]. Natural orifice transluminal endoscopic surgery (NOTES) is currently of major research interest as it may offer significant clinical potential for endoscopic procedures in the future, although many further issues are still unresolved. The application of this concept to surgical oncology is already common practice in certain fields such as the rectum [2], while it still needs to be thoroughly investigated in many others.

Esophagus

Technology seemed to lend a hand to surgery when in 1989 Gerhard Buess presented his mediastinoscope [3]. Introduced through a cervical incision, it allowed dissection of the esophagus under videoscopic visualization. Despite the report in small series of a consistent benefit in terms of a decrease in respiratory complications in terms of both thoracotomy and the transhiatal approach, today the technique has almost been abandoned.

Two minimally invasive techniques continue to be performed in specialized centers:

M. Morino (✉)
Centre of Mini-Invasive Surgery, S. Giovanni Battista University Hospital, Turin, Italy

New Technologies in Surgical Oncology. Antonio Mussa (Ed.)
© Springer-Verlag Italia 2010

the three-stage operation by right thoracoscopy and laparoscopy, and the transhiatal laparoscopic approach. The three-stage intervention has been proposed in consistent series by Akaishi [4], Nguyen [5] and Dexter [6]. They have all demonstrated feasibility of the technique in a reasonable operating time, but results with respect to morbidity and mortality were contradictory, as in the first two series functional results showed an improvement, while in the third they remained as high as for radical thoracotomic dissection. In order to limit the rate of complications other minimally invasive techniques for esophagectomy have been proposed in the same years. Transhiatal esophagectomy was first described by DePaula in 1995 [7], followed by other reports [8,9]. This approach has proven feasible and safe in the medium-term follow-up, at least for distal cancers.

Recently the scientific world started to investigate the frontier of NOTES also applied to the mediastinum. The experience till now is restricted to the animal model in order to understand the feasibility of different techniques. A first report from the Homerton University Hospital of London [10] tested transesophageal lymph node removal in surviving pigs together with a number of other mediastinal procedures. In all cases the access was performed with the aid of endoscopic ultrasound (EUS) and closed with conventional endoclips. Although feasibility was proven, the technique proved challenging. Sacrifice at 6 weeks showed in all cases a well-healed esophageal incision with no signs of mediastinitis, although the endoclips allowed only closure of the mucosal layer. To limit the risks of a leakage the same group and others [11] tested the benefit of tunnelling the transesophageal access inside the submucosal layer for about 10 cm, although this made the procedure evidently more complex. When safety of the access-site sealing is assessed as reliable in survival studies, the transesophageal route could be considered an easier, reproducible alternative to access the mediastinum [12].

Stomach

Western countries still experience a large majority of advanced lesions at primary diagnosis, limiting any application of minimally invasive concepts, to respect oncological criteria. In fact, today the role for laparoscopic treatment is reserved to T1-2/N0 gastric cancer [13].

Flexible endoscopy already plays a major role in the treatment of early stage disease. Endoscopic mucosal resection (EMR) and endoscopic submucosal dissection (ESD) are advanced techniques and may be considered the ultimate 'minimally' invasive treatments for early stage cancers, such as selected T1/N0 adenocarcinoma (see Chapter 10). Therefore, NOTES may initially have a role in furthering the application of such endeavors to slightly more advanced stages. In fact, it may ensure oncological providence in the treatment of those T1 lesions with higher risk of lymphatic metastases which currently are advised to lie beyond the range of pure endoscopic resection for reasons of oncological propriety rather than technical capacity. NOTES could supplement ESD by providing for direct sampling of sentinel nodes from the perigastric lymph basin. Subsequently perhaps a NOTES technique may develop which is capable of performing full-thickness wedge resections for T2/N0 adenocarcinomas. In fact Kaehler has already successfully performed the technique in a clinical setting by using of a flexible stapling system (SurgAssist™, Power Medical Interventions, Germany) [14] on two patients, one with an early cancer and one with a carcinoid tumor, obtaining a full-thickness resection of the gastric wall under gastroscopic control and retrieving specimens up to 4 cm x 4 cm in size. A similar technique could be proposed with even more clear indication for the treatment of gastrointestinal stromal tumors (GIST), which are rare neoplasms with a "potential malignancy" difficult to assess preoperatively [15].

Recently, a growing number of clinical trials evaluating the feasibility and accuracy of sentinel lymph node biopsy in gastric cancer have been published [16–18]. However, the lymphatic drainage of the stomach is considerably more complex than that of ectodermal organs like the breast and skin due to their complex embryological development. Therefore, the application of the sentinel lymph node concept in gastric cancer is still under discussion. Although the accuracy and reliability of sentinel node navigation is similar at least in selected centres [19,20], this theory has yet to be definitively proven. Furthermore, it is known that lymphatic mapping becomes less accurate as the disease advances. Therefore it proves more reliable when applied to those stages most suitable for endoscopic resective techniques [19]. In those cases NOTES may provide a complement for endoscopic sentinel node biopsy and an oncological supplement to current EMR/ESD techniques. The technical feasibility of lymphatic mapping and sentinel node biopsy by NOTES for the stomach in a pig model has already been proven [21].

Further investigation is required to comprehend the feasibility and applicability of intraoperative analysis of the sentinel nodes.

Colon and Rectum

For a long time colorectal surgeons seemed immune to the contagious excitement which surrounded the development of laparoscopic surgery throughout the 1980s and 1990s, ignoring or even rejecting the unique patient benefits. Colorectal surgery lagged behind, as the challenges of working in multiple quadrants with the need for extensive vascular control within an often thick friable mesentery, the requirement of anastomosis, and the surgical indications such as inflammatory bowel disease and neoplasia dampened enthusiasm [22]. Reports of port site metastases further decelerated the adoption of the techniques and the penetration of the procedures [23]. Finally, only after the COST trial was presented at the May 2004 meeting of the American Society of Colon and Rectal Surgeons and simultaneously published in the New England Journal of Medicine [24] did acceptance accelerate.

Today laparoscopy has actually proven to be the most important advance also in colorectal surgery since the introduction of surgical stapling [25]. Oncologic safety has now been demonstrated for laparoscopy-assisted surgery for colon adenocarcinoma after 3 and 5 years of follow-up. Pooled data from large multicentre and smaller single-centre trials demonstrate that the modality conveys significant short-term benefits as compared with open surgery, although the full potential has probably not yet been reached. Currently, the data supports improvements in wound morbidity, intraoperative blood loss, narcotic analgesia requirements, time to resumption of bowel movements, and time to discharge from hospital. There is a large potential for improved short-term results when combined with current and developing enhanced-recovery programmes. For rectal cancer, the role of laparoscopic surgery is less clear. Data from the first large multicentre trial [26] suggest that laparoscopic dissection may compromise the circumferential resection margin, and this issue will be the focus of ongoing and planned trials. Certain short-term benefits have been shown in pooled analyses of smaller non-randomized trials [27,28], such as a decrease in overall morbidity and a marked reduction of duration of postoperative hospital stay.

Since the demonstration of a benefit of MIS applied to colon cancer treatment, patients, surgeons, and industrial partners have begun the quest for the next paradigm shift. The debate began between the opportunity of single port access or single incision access surgery [29] or a NOTES approach [30,31].

In truth, NOTES was already familiar to all colorectal surgeons thanks to the efforts of Gerhard Buess who pioneered and disseminated to the world transanal endoscopic microsurgery (TEM) [32], which can be clearly considered a direct ancestor in the lineage to NOTES in the field of general surgery.

On the one hand the slow adoption of laparoscopy and on the other familiarity with TEM together have led to the interesting development of transanal specimen extraction and anastomosis techniques. Numerous surgeons have described and demonstrated both the technical aspects and the results [33,34].

The same concepts on the role of NOTES in sentinel node biopsy as already illustrated for gastric cancer can be potentially applied to the colorectal district as well. Some interesting work in this field has been recently reported [35]. As for gastric cancer, flexible endoscopy techniques (EMR/ESD) represent a standard for early cancers not invading the submucosal layer and therefore at low risk for N+. Moreover, the concept interests Western countries much more due to the increased incidence of this kind of disease, which is expected to increase even more now that screening programs are beginning all around. Even for the colorectal district a transgastric NOTES technique was described after tests on an animal model. The sigmoid colon was fully exposed by an intracolonic magnet under extracorporeal control. Colonoscopy facilitated submucosal injection of methylene blue dye (3 mL) at the apex of the sigmoid loop under direct transgastric vision. The mesocolon was searched for blue-stained lymph channels and nodes, the latter being resected and retrieved by the intraperitoneal endoscope. Each procedure was a technical success proving that sentinel node biopsy can be performed without abdominal wall transgression.

The potential clinical benefit which patients may accrue from targeted dissection as definitive treatment in place of radical operation has not yet been definitively proven, but it may be considerable at least in the short-term. However, oncological propriety and outcomes must be maintained. In particular, methods by which regional nodal staging can be assured if standard operation is avoided still need to be established. Sentinel node mapping is one such putative means of doing so which deserves serious consideration from this perspective as it performs a similar function for breast cancer and melanoma and because there is already considerable evidence to suggest that the technique in colonic neoplasia may be at its most accurate in germinal disease. In addition, it may already be employed by laparoscopy while solely transluminal means of its deployment are advancing. While the confluence of operative technologies and techniques now coming on-stream has the potential to precipitate a dramatic shift in the paradigm for the management of early stage colonic neoplasia, considerable confirmatory study is required to ensure that oncology propriety and treatment efficacy is maintained so that patient benefit may be maximised.

Nevertheless, the present application of NOTES to the colon and rectum district is represented by transvaginal minilaparoscopic-assisted natural orifice surgery (MA-NOS) for radical sigmoidectomy. A preliminary experience on humans consisting of four selected patients has recently been reported [36]. In order to maintain triangulation the surgeon is positioned at the right side of the patient and uses the transvaginal trocar for dissection and stapling of both the inferior mesenteric vessels and the upper rectum. The colonic resection is then performed extracorporeally and is followed by an intra-abdominal endoscopically assisted stapled anastomosis. Although the authors report that all oncological principles governing resection and management of the clinical situation were accomplished, the report raised several concerns. We can say that transvaginal MA-NOS sigmoidectomy is a feasible procedure. Follow-up will give us data on the oncological results of the technique.

Transanal Endoscopic Microsurgery

Twenty-five years ago, the introduction of transanal endoscopic microsurgery (TEM) apparently made possible the combination of the advantages of a less invasive transanal approach with low recurrence rates due to enhanced visualization of the surgical field allowing a more precise dissection. TEM was initially proposed as a technique for excision of benign rectal neoplasms. Later, indications were extended to "low risk" pT1 rectal adenocarcinomas [37] with curative intent [38] and more invasive rectal adenocarcinomas for palliative purposes. To date, only one randomized study [39] has compared the outcome of anterior resection (26 patients) and TEM (24 patients) for T1 rectal tumors. At a mean follow-up of 46 months, local recurrence (4%) and 5-year survival (96%) rates were similar in the two groups. These data suggest that TEM may offer some advantages in respect to anterior resection for T1 tumors, with similar oncological results. Patients with T1 tumors with favorable pathological features may undergo local excision alone with acceptable oncological outcomes [40], whereas those with unfavorable criteria require radical surgery or adjuvant treatment [41]. More recently, several authors [42–45] have proposed a combination of preoperative radio-chemotherapy with local resection by TEM with radical intent for pT2 tumors.

We have recently reported of a retrospective analysis of a prospective consecutive series representing probably the largest experience reported of patients with benign and malignant rectal tumors excised by TEM [46]. Our analysis confirms that the procedure is safe, affected by low postoperative mortality and morbidity rates. In the present study, only 23/300 patients (7.7%) experienced minor complications and no mortality occurred. This confirms several previous reports in which complication rate ranged between 2 and 30% [38,47–50] The most common local complications were bleeding and dehiscence or fistula.

The standard indication for TEM with curative intent is the treatment of adenomas and pT1 neoplasms of the rectum. With these indications we scored a recurrence rate of 11/222 (4.9%) which is comparable to smaller series appearing in the literature. Other authors have compared TEM to transanal local excision according to Parks. Local excision was found to be affected by a higher recurrence rate ranging between 10 and 27% [50–52]. The higher recurrence risk of conventional transanal surgery compared to TEM is certainly due to the lower rate of complete excision with tumor-free margins [50,53–55] in conventionally treated patients.

A key point for obtaining satisfactory results with TEM is the appropriate selection of patients. A precise evaluation of the depth of tumor invasion and lymph node metastasis is crucial. No recurrence was observed till now among the 38 pT1 cancers confirmed at histology in our series [46]. Other authors report of a risk of recurrence and metastatic spread if oncological criteria are not fully matched. Histopathological criteria which are important predictors of lymph node metastasis include incomplete resection margins, invasion of the submucosa (sm2-3), poorly differentiated histology and lymphovascular invasion [56–59].

TEM has been proposed as a technology to be used for NOTES. Entry into the peritoneal cavity during a resection of rectosigmoid lesions has been described, and safe closure can be obtained. The group of Portland (USA) recently reported on the feasibility both on animal models and human cadavers of transrectal NOTES procedures by using TEM instrumentation [60]. They also reported several challenges for bridging to human clinical use. In fact, TEM instruments are currently designed for intraluminal tasks low in the pelvis, with 5-mm to 10-mm port sizes. For this reason Gerhard Buess is now working to a newly designed instrumentarium derived from the original TEM device, consisting of specially designed instruments and a single-port technique, to allow abdominal surgery with rigid instruments under the principles of NOTES [61].

Final Considerations

The American Society of Colon and Rectal Surgeons and the Society of American Gastrointestinal Endoscopic Surgeons stated that "laparoscopic colectomy for curable cancer results in equivalent survival compared to open colectomy when performed by experienced surgeons" [62]. On the other hand, further data regarding other districts, such as the esophagus, stomach and rectum are needed before any definitive conclusions can be reached.

The arrival of these data is being accompanied by a new objective, represented by a further improvement in the reduction of invasiveness. Nevertheless, NOTES in oncology and other areas is associated with numerous technical and ethical questions. The American Society of Gastrointestinal Endoscopy and the Society of American Gastrointestinal Endoscopic Surgery have convened a working group, NOSCAR, to formulate guidelines so as to move this concept in a safe, collaborative and ethical manner. Similar measures have been taken by the European Association for Endoscopic Surgery and the European Society of Gastrointestinal Endoscopy by joining the EURONOTES Foundation. The goal is to move further by combining the technically feasible EMR/ESD endoluminal resection of T1 cancers with unfavorable characteristics for increased risk of lymph nodes metastases after sentinel node transluminal sampling. The newborn EURONOTES Clinical Registry (www.euronotes.world.it) will help us to address all the ongoing issues, and understand which role NOTES will play also in surgical oncology in the near future.

While all this is being investigated, TEM, which can be clearly considered a direct ancestor in the lineage to NOTES in the field of general surgery, continues to contribute with its clinical application, to a real minimally invasive technique for early rectal cancers.

Mini-Invasive Thoracic Techniques in Oncological Surgery

Mini-invasive techniques can be used in oncological surgery with thoracic-pulmonary pathologies.

The evaluation of the area extension of the primary bronchopulmonary cancer is helped by radiological diagnosis (CT, RMN, PET), endoscopic diagnosis (bronchoscopy), surgical diagnosis (mediastinoscopy, mediastinotomy, supraclavicular biopsy, thoracoscopy).

The thoracoscopy was introduced by Jacobaeus in 1913 as therapy for patients suffering from tubercular disease and was used until the 1950s to dissect pleural adhesions in order to promote lung collapse during the execution of the therapeutic pneumothorax as proposed by Forlanini. In 1990, diagnostic thoracoscopy became therapeutic and acquired the name of video assisted thoracic surgery (VATS).

VATS offers the possibility of mini-invasive surgery, using a particular endoscopic instrument and a mini fiber-optic camera to perform thoracic surgery with reduced surgical trauma due to access; it also reduces post-operative pain in comparison with traditional surgical techniques. VATS allows a prompt mobilization of the patient and reduces hospital stays. Due to the fact that it is less invasive than traditional techniques, VATS also allows the performance of surgery in patients suffering from serious respiratory insufficiency that might otherwise result in a contraindication to the operation.

The mini-invasive technique used in thoracic surgery has a few simplifications in comparison with abdominal surgery, since the trocars used allow free passage of the instruments with no need for any valvular apparatus. In fact the pneumothorax, whether provoked by surgically performed pleurotomies or favored by the anesthetist via selective pulmonary ventilation, facilitates surgery in the collapsed pulmonary parenchyma and the parietal, mediastinal and diaphragmatic pleura. Unlike the case of abdominal surgery, there is no need to restore the pneumothorax. For this reason the thoracoscopy column has no carbon dioxide insufflator, since the chest maintains its normal expansion thanks to the mechanical action performed by the ribs, with no need for the mechanical action of gas.

Thoracic surgery using the mini-invasive method was first proposed for the treatment of relapsing spontaneous pneumothorax.

VATS in Oncological Surgery

Oncological surgery in the pleura making use of VATS includes pleural biopsies, pleurectomies and the removal of neurinomas of the intercostal nerves. Together with these abscission procedures, thoracoscopy can also be used to insufflate talc into the pleural cavity in order to determine chemical pleurisy and treat patients suffering from relapsing pleural effusion which cannot be treated with other therapies.

VATS can be considered as complementary therapy to mediastinoscopy and mediastinotomy in the diagnosis of mediastinal adenopathies since there are some anatomical areas which can be investigated only via thoracoscopic access. In fact, hilar subcarinal adenopathies of the posterior mediastinum can be diagnosed and treated with thoracoscopies.

Oncological surgery in the lungs with mini-invasive methods includes the removal of pulmonary nodules via atypical resections of the pulmonary parenchyma and abscission of primary and secondary lung neoplasms by performing pulmonary segmental and lobar resections.

The resection of the pulmonary parenchyma in cases of lung neoplasms must always be associated with pulmonary and mediastinal lymphadenectomy, which makes it possible to correctly divide the neoplastic disease into stages.

The ideal candidates for pulmonary resection via thoracoscopy are patients who are carriers of a small peripheral pulmonary neoplasm, growing out of the visceral pleura and confined in the inferior lobe.

The limitations of the technique are the impossibility of manual palpation of the pulmonary parenchyma which in open surgery makes it possible to establish the extension of the parenchymal resection.

Other disadvantages of VATS in comparison with conventional techniques are extended length of surgery, the risk of severe intra-operative hemorrhages which can force a thoracotomy, the possibility of tumor dissemination, the necessity to perform a small thoracotomy to extract the surgical specimen.

VATS has several advantages over traditional techniques. It is less invasive and therefore there are fewer days of hospitalization, fewer symptoms of pain and limited esthetic damage. Thanks to the use of the endoscopic instruments and the fiber-optic camera to magnify vision, it is also possible to perform high-precision surgery in areas that would be hard to access using traditional methods.

References

1. Kalloo AN, Singh VK, Jagannath SB et al (2004) Flexible transgastric peritoneoscopy: a novel approach to diagnostic and therapeutic interventions in the peritoneal cavity. Gastrointest Endosc 60:114–117

2. Buess G, Kipfmüller K, Ibald R et al (1989) Transanal endoscopic microsurgery in rectal cancer. Chirurg 60:901–904

3. Kipfmüller K, Buess G, Naruhn M, Bätz W (1990) Endoscopic-microsurgical dissection of the esophagus. An animal experiment study. Chirurg 61:187–191

4. Akaishi T, Kaneda I, Higuchi N et al (1996) Thoracoscopic en bloc total esophagectomy with radical mediastinal lymphadenectomy. J Thorac Cardiovasc Surg 112:1533–1540; discussion 1540–1541

5. Nguyen NT, Follette DM, Wolfe BM et al (2000) Comparison of minimally invasive esophagectomy with transthoracic and transhiatal esophagectomy. Arch Surg 135:920–925

6. Dexter SP, Martin IG, McMahon MJ (1996) Radical thoracoscopic esophagectomy for cancer. Surg Endosc 10:147–151

7. DePaula AL, Hashiba K, Ferreira EA et al (1995) Laparoscopic transhiatal esophagectomy with esophagogastroplasty. Surg Laparosc Endosc 5:1–5

8. Swanstrom LL, Hansen P (1997) Laparoscopic total esophagectomy. Arch Surg 132:943–947; discussion 947–949

9. Bonavina L, Bona D, Binyom PR, Peracchia A (2004) A laparoscopy-assisted surgical approach to esophageal carcinoma. J Surg Res 117:52–57

10. Fritscher-Ravens A, Patel K, Ghanbari A et al (2007) Natural orifice transluminal endoscopic surgery (NOTES) in the mediastinum: long-term survival animal experiments in transesophageal access, including minor surgical procedures. Endoscopy 39:870–875

11. Willingham FF, Gee DW, Lauwers GY et al (2008) Natural orifice transesophageal mediastinoscopy and thoracoscopy. Surg Endosc 22:1042–1047

12. Perretta S, Allemann P, Dallemagne B, Marescaux J (2009) Natural orifice transluminal endoscopic surgery (NOTES) for neoplasia of the chest and mediastinum. Surg Oncol 18:177–180

13. Shiraishi N, Yasuda K, Kitano S (2006) Laparoscopic gastrectomy with lymph node dissection for gastric cancer. Gastric Cancer 167–176

14. Kaehler G, Grobholz R, Langner C et al (2006) A new technique of endoscopic full-thickness resection using a flexible stapler. Endoscopy 38:86–89

15. Dholakia C, Gould J (2008) Minimally invasive resection of gastrointestinal stromal tumors. Surg Clin North Am 88:1009–1018

16. Aikou T, Kitagawa Y, Kitajima M (2006) Sentinel lymph node mapping with GI cancer. Cancer Metastasis Rev 25:269–277

17. Kitagawa Y, Kitajima M (2006) Diagnostic validity of radio-guided sentinel node mapping for gastric cancer: a review of current status and future direction. Surg Technol Int 15:32–36

18. Ishigami S, Natsugoe S, Uenosono Y et al (2007) Usefulness of sentinel node biopsy in laparoscopic partial gastrectomy for early gastric cancer. Hepatogastroenterology 54:2164–2166

19. Saikawa Y, Otani Y, Kitagawa Y et al (2006) Interim results of sentinel node biopsy during laparoscopic gastrectomy: possible role in function-preserving surgery for early cancer. World J Surg 30:1962–1968

20. Kitagawa Y, Fujii H, Mukai M et al (2002) Radio-guided sentinel node detection for gastric cancer. Br J Surg 89:604–608

21. Cahill RA, Asakuma M, Perretta S et al (2009) Gastric lymphatic mapping for sentinel node biopsy by natural orifice transluminal endoscopic surgery (NOTES). Surg Endosc 23:1110–1116

22. Wexner SD, Johansen OB (1992) Laparoscopic bowel resection: advantages and limitations. Ann Med 24:105–110

23. Wexner SD, Cohen SM (1995) Port site metastases after laparoscopic colorectal surgery for cure of malignancy. Br J Surg 82:295–298

24. Clinical Outcomes of Surgical Therapy Study Group (2004) A comparison of laparoscopically assisted and open colectomy for colon cancer. N Engl J Med 350:2050–2059

25. Ravitch MM, Steichen FM, Fishbein RH et al (1964) Clinical experiences with the soviet mechanical bronchus stapler (UKB-25). J Thorac Cardiovasc Surg 47:446–454

26. Jayne DG, Guillou PJ, Thorpe H et al (2007) Randomized trial of laparoscopic-assisted resection of colorectal carcinoma: 3-year results of the UK MRC CLASICC Trial Group. J Clin Oncol 25:3061–3068

27. Morino M, Allaix ME, Giraudo G et al (2005) Laparoscopic versus open surgery for extraperitoneal rectal cancer: a prospective comparative study. Surg Endosc 19:1460–1467

28. Feliciotti F, Guerrieri M, Paganini AM et al (2003) Long-term results of laparoscopic versus open resections for rectal cancer for 124 unselected patients. Surg Endosc 17:1530–1535

29. Leroy J, Cahill RA, Peretta S, Marescaux J (2008) Single port sigmoidectomy in an experimental model with survival. Surg Innov 15:260–265

30. Whiteford MH, Denk PM, Swanström LL (2007) Feasibility of radical sigmoid colectomy performed as natural orifice translumenal endoscopic surgery (NOTES) using transanal endoscopic microsurgery. Surg Endosc 21:1870–1874

31. Leroy J, Cahill RA, Perretta S et al (2009) Natural orifice translumenal endoscopic surgery (NOTES) applied totally to sigmoidectomy: an original technique with survival in a porcine model. Surg Endosc 23:24–30

32. Buess G (1991) Transanal microsurgery. Langenbecks Arch Chir Suppl Kongressbd 441–447

33. Sylla P, Willingham FF, Sohn DK et al (2008) NOTES rectosigmoid resection using transanal endoscopic microsurgery (TEM) with transgastric endoscopic assistance: a pilot study in swine. J Gastrointest Surg 12:1717–1723

34. Franklin ME Jr, Kelley H, Kelley M et al (2008) Transvaginal extraction of the specimen after total laparoscopic right hemicolectomy with intracorporeal anastomosis. Surg Laparosc Endosc Percutan Tech 18:294–298

35. Cahill RA, Perretta S, Leroy J et al (2008) Lymphatic mapping and sentinel node biopsy in the colonic mesentery by natural orifice transluminal endoscopic surgery (NOTES). Ann Surg Oncol 15:2677–2683

36. Lacy AM, Delgado S, Rojas OA (2008) MA-NOS radical sigmoidectomy: report of a transvaginal resection in the human. Surg Endosc 22:1717–1723

37. Hermanek P, Gall FP (1986) Early (microinvasive) colorectal carcinoma. Pathology, diagnosis, surgical treatment. Int J Colorectal Dis 1:79–84

38. Mentges B, Buess G, Raestrup H et al (1994) TEM results of the Tuebingen group. Endosc Surg Allied Technol 2:247–250

39. Winde G, Nottberg H, Keller R et al (1996) Surgical cure for early rectal carcinomas (T1). Transanal endoscopic microsurgery vs. anterior resection. Dis Colon Rectum 39:969–976

40. Floyd ND, Saclarides TJ (2006) Transanal endoscopic microsurgical resection of pT1 rectal tumors. Dis Colon Rectum 49:164–168

41. Bentrem DJ, Okabe S, Wong WD et al (2005) T1 adenocarcinoma of the rectum: transanal excision or radical surgery? Ann Surg 242:472–477

42. Lezoche E, Guerrieri M, Paganini AM, Feliciotti F (2002) Long-term results of patients with pT2 rectal cancer treated with radiotherapy and transanal endoscopic microsurgical excision. World J Surg 26:1170–1174

43. Borschitz T, Heintz A, Junginger T (2007) Transanal endoscopic microsurgical excision of pT2 rectal cancer: results and possible indications. Dis Colon Rectum 50:292–301

44. Duek SD, Issa N, Hershko DD, Krausz MM (2008) Outcome of transanal endoscopic microsurgery and adjuvant radiotherapy in patients with T2 rectal cancer. Dis Colon Rectum 51:379–384; discussion 384

45. Tjandra T (2006) Long-term results in patients with T2–3 N0 distal rectal cancer undergoing radiotherapy before transanal endoscopic microsurgery. Tech Coloproctol 10:158
46. Allaix ME, Arezzo A, Caldart M et al (in press, Festa F. Morino M. Transanal Endoscopic Microsurgery for rectal neoplasms. Experience of 300 consecutive cases. Dis Colon Rectum, in press
47. Stipa F, Lucandri G, Ferri M et al (2004) Local excision of rectal cancer with transanal endoscopic microsurgery (TEM). Anticancer Res 24:1167–1172
48. Lezoche E, Guerrieri M, Paganini AM et al (1996) Is transanal endoscopic microsurgery (TEM) a valid treatment for rectal tumors? Surg Endosc 10:736–741
49. Heintz A, Morshel M, Junginger T (1998) Comparison of results afer transanal endoscopic microsurgery and radical resection for T1 carcinoma of the rectum. Surg Endosc 12:1145–1148
50. Middleton PF, Sutherland LM, Maddern GJ (2005) Transanal endoscopic microsurgery: a systematic review. Dis Colon Rectum 48:270–284
51. Lee W, Lee D, Choi S, Chun H (2003) Transanal endoscopic microsurgery and radical surgery for T1 and T2 rectal cancer. Surg Endosc 17:1283–1287
52. Langer C, Liersch T, Suss M et al (2003) Surgical cure for early rectal carcinoma and large adenoma: Transanal endoscopic microsurgery (using ultrasound or electrosurgery) compared to conventional local and radical resection. Int J Colorectal Dis 18:222–229
53. Sakamoto GD, MacKeigan JM, Senagore AJ (1991) Transanal excision of large, rectal villous adenomas. Dis Colon Rectum 34:880–885
54. Gavagan JA, Whiteford MH, Swanstrom LL (2004) Full-thickness intraperitoneal excision by transanal endoscopic microsurgery does not increase short-term complications. Am J Surg 187:630–634
55. Steele RJC, Hershman MJ, Mortensen NJM et al (1996) Transanal endoscopic microsurgery – initial experience from three centres in the United Kingdom. Br J Surg 83:207–210
56. Nascimbeni R, Burgart LJ, Nivatvongs S, Larson DR (2002) Risk of lymph node metastasis in T1 carcinoma of the colon and rectum. Dis Colon Rectum 45:200–206
57. Brodsky JT, Richard GK, Cohen AM, Minsky BD (1992) Variables correlated with the risk of lymph node metastasis in early rectal cancer. Cancer 69:322–326
58. Blumberg D, Paty PB, Guillem JG et al (1999) All patients with small intramural rectal cancers are at risk for lymph node metastasis. Dis Colon Rectum 42:881–885
59. Paty PB, Nash GM, Baron GM et al (2002) Long-term results of local excision for rectal cancer. Ann Surg 236:522–529
60. Denk PM, Swanström LL, Whiteford MH (2008) Transanal endoscopic microsurgical platform for natural orifice surgery. Gastrointest Endosc 68:954–959
61. Buess G, Becerra-Garcia F, Misra MC (2008) Instruments for transluminal laparoscopic surgery or "NOTES". Minim Invasive Ther Allied Technol 17:331–335
62. Cera S, Wexner SD (2005) Minimally invasive treatment of colon cancer. Cancer J 11:26–35

Radioguided Surgery in Oncological Surgery

3

S. Sandrucci, R. Moscato, L. Matera, A. Galetto

The concept of radioguided surgery involves the use of a radiation detection probe system for the intraoperative detection of radionuclides. The use of gamma detection probe technology in radioguided surgery has expanded tremendously and has evolved into what is now considered an established discipline within the practice of surgery, revolutionizing the surgical management of many malignancies, including breast cancer, melanoma and colorectal cancer. The specific application of mono-clonal antibodies to radioguided surgery has been the basis for the development of *radioimmunoguided surgery*; the use of oncotrophic or lymphotrophic tracers is the basic principle of *radioguided surgery*.

Radioimmunoguided Surgery

In the mid-1970s, crucial advances in immunology led to widespread fascination with the development of radiolabelled antibodies for immunoscintigraphy of primary or secondary tumors. The availability of these radiolabelled tumor-seeking agents constituted the first step toward radioimmunoguided surgery [1] in patients with colorectal cancer. Shortly thereafter, some research groups began exploring the diagnostic potential of radioimmunodetection, a new technique that combined the administration of radiolabelled antibodies with external imaging to identify clinically occult tumors.

Other groups examined the potential of intraoperative radioactivity counting to detect the uptake of radiolabelled MABs by malignant cells. These latter experiences led to the development of a dedicated handheld gamma-detecting probe for intraoperative use, which improved the sensitivity of external radioimmunodetection.

S. Sandrucci (✉)
Surgical Oncology Unit, S. Giovanni Battista University Hospital, Turin, Italy

New Technologies in Surgical Oncology. Antonio Mussa (Ed.)
© Springer-Verlag Italia 2010

In the early 1990s, the development of second-generation MABs specifically for colon cancer led to further improvements in radioimmunoguided surgery for patients with this malignancy. Subsequent pilot clinical studies revealed efficient tumor localization in 86% of patients with primary colorectal cancer and 97% of patients with recurrent disease. In several cases, intraoperative use of the gamma probe with CC49 led to the modification of the planned operative procedure, thus impacting decision making. These encouraging findings indicated that the application of radioimmunoguided surgery in patients with primary or recurrent colorectal cancer might yield clinically relevant information regarding the pattern of disease, thus challenging the adequacy of the traditional procedure alone for adoptive cellular immunotherapy. Moreover, immunohistochemical staining of radioimmunoguided surgery-positive lymph nodes with anti-cytokeratin MABs increases the likelihood of identifying occult tumor cells in these nodes.

Although the conceptually simple technique of radioimmunoguided surgery has been investigated and refined for almost 30 years, it still has inherent limitations. The poor availability of specific MABs has been overcome only in selected cases, such as colorectal cancer; in the majority of tumors, the efficacy of radioimmunoguided surgery remains uncertain. Other critical issues, such as choice of the radionuclide to label the MAB, are still controversial. Therefore, the initial enthusiasm generated by early results with radioimmunoguided surgery has been dampened in the past decade. Growing knowledge of antigen-antibody relationships and the development of new and superior tumor-targeting agents might constitute the basis for future advances with radioimmunoguided surgery.

Radioguided Surgery

Breast

The widespread use of mammography has increased the detection of preinvasive cancers; many authors indicate that 15 to 25% of diagnosed breast cancers are intraductal carcinomas, most of which are clinically occult. A non-palpable breast lesion can be localized by injecting carbon particles or by inserting a hooked wire under mammographic or ultrasound guidance, although both techniques have shortcomings. Carbon particles in the surgically removed tissue can render histological evaluation of the specimen problematic. During insertion of a hooked wire, the needle introducing the wire may become displaced. Attempting to remove and reinsert the wire is unlikely to be successful and will increase the risk of bleeding and hematoma.

Radioguided occult lesion localization was pioneered in 1996 at the European Institute of Oncology in Milan (Italy) for localizing non-palpable breast lesions. This method marked a natural evolution from earlier studies on radioguided sentinel node biopsy for breast carcinoma. Increasing success and enthusiasm for the sentinel node technique generated great expectations among surgeons of this institute for the potential of nuclear medicine to solve other problems, such as preoperative localization of occult or non-palpable breast lesions. The non-palpable breast lesion is injected under stereotactic guidance using large-size radiolabelled particles (such as those used in lung perfusion scintigraphy) to ensure that the radiotracer would not move from the injection site, and the lesion removed surgically on the following day. The gamma probe proved just as effective in assisting intraoperative localization and removal here, as in sentinel node biopsy. When compared to wire localization, it provides better centering of the lesion within the specimen and reduces the amount of healthy tissue removed. Most importantly, it provides the surgeon with a quick and simple means of locating and removing the lesion in the operating room. The absence of side effects or complications also contributes to its success [2,3].

However, radioguided occult lesion localization should not be attempted in women with diffuse microcalcifications and multifocal or multicentric lesions. Moreover, the technique requires close collaboration between the radiologist, the nuclear physician, the surgeon, and the pathologist. A team learning curve of 30 procedures is sufficient for the correct execution of each step of the procedure. The best results are obtained when the lesion is localized under ultrasonography guidance; this procedure is simple and fast (5–10 min maximum), with excellent correspondence between location of the hot spot and the lesion's position. The echogenicity changes caused by the presence of both the needle and tracer make it possible to verify that the needle tip is inserted into the lesion and that the tracer is correctly injected.

More problematic and complex is the approach using x-ray stereotaxis. The injection needle is not always inserted to the correct depth. The distance between the injected radiopaque spot and the lesion must always be checked on the standard mammogram taken after injection. Centring very superficial lesions is difficult, while another problem is lesions in the central quadrant of the breast, where the probability of injecting the tracer in a galactophore is high. Macroaggregates of albumin do not move from the injection site, and there is no diffusion in the breast tissue around the lesion, provided that the radiotracer has not been introduced into the lymphatic vessels or galactophorous ducts. This allows a large lapse of time prior to surgery, consistent with physical decay of 99mTc.

Parathyroid

In the experience of Norman and colleagues from the University of South Florida [4] the cause of primary hyperparathyroidism is a single adenoma in 95% of cases. In the opinion of these authors, the use of physiological measures of parathyroid gland activity and the assessment of PTH production (directly or indirectly) in the operating theatre is responsible for this more accurate accounting of the number of true single adenomas.

It is now generally acknowledged that high-quality scintigraphy with 99mTc-sestamibi can accurately localize parathyroid adenomas in 85 to 95% of patients with primary hyperparathyroidism. The addition of single photon emission computed tomography (SPECT) imaging considerably improves the localization of particular ectopic sites otherwise difficult to explore, such as the retro-esophageal space or mediastinum. Any imaging protocol based on the use of 99mTc-sestamibi intrinsically implies scinti-

graphic exploration not only of the neck (where parathyroid adenomas are most frequently located, reflecting the normal anatomy of the parathyroid glands), but also of
the entire chest to rule out the possible presence of tumors in ectopic locations. A
wealth of information currently supports the use of 99mTc-sestamibi scintigraphy as a
preoperative localization technique for unilateral neck exploration and minimally invasive radioguided parathyroidectomy [5]. In patients with hyperparathyroidism, any
parathyroid gland that is physiologically or supraphysiologically active and synthesiz-
ing hormone will become radioactive after the injection of 99mTc-sestamibi, while
those that are dormant do not. In Norman's opinion, the most important aspect of radioguided parathyroid surgery is not only the use of a gamma probe to help the surgeon
find the overproducing parathyroid gland, but also the estimation of how much hormone any individual parathyroid gland is producing, based on metabolic activity as
mirrored by the uptake of 99mTc-sestamibi. This indicates when the patient is cured
and the operation can be concluded. In this regard, Norman believes the gamma probe
can distinguish the difference between a normal parathyroid gland, a hyperplastic
parathyroid gland, and a parathyroid adenoma. In fact, the probe is so accurate at this
determination that frozen sections were necessary in a minority of Norman's cases
(only 2.2% of their last 3,000 parathyroid operations).

Gamma-probe guidance enables the surgeon to perform a rather small skin incision,
improved cosmesis being one of the main advantages of this technique, which can also
be performed under local anesthesia. The operating time is reduced compared to that
for conventional exploration not based on radioguidance, and the patient can be dis-
charged from the hospital earlier. As with other radioguided surgical procedures, the
technique requires that the whole team involved (nuclear medicine specialist, surgeon,
pathologist, nursing staff) achieve a satisfactory amount of experience and smooth
interaction among team members. Some recommendations should be followed when
considering minimally invasive radioguided parathyroidectomy: (1) the most accurate
preoperative scintigraphic modality available should be used, possibly dual-tracer sub-
traction scintigraphy or dual-phase 99mTc-sestamibi SPECT; (2) both in vivo and ex
vivo gamma probe counting should be obtained to evaluate the success and completeness of the surgery; (3) radiation exposure to the surgeon and operating room person-
nel should be minimized by administering the lowest dose of 99mTc-sestamibi proved
to be effective for performing minimally invasive radioguided parathyroidectomy.
Intraoperative quick PTH measurement appears to be strictly related to the minimally
invasive radioguided parathyroidectomy protocol used. The operating surgeon, however, must realize that new techniques and tools are not a substitute for experience, and
having a probe in the operating room does not necessarily make an expert out of a surgeon who sees parathyroid patients infrequently. Common sense and a thorough knowledge of parathyroid anatomy are critically important.

Neuroendocrine Tumors

For patients with localized disease, surgery remains the treatment of choice. In
patients with metastatic carcinoids presenting with liver and mesenteric metastases,

conservative resections of the intestine, mesenteric tumors, and fibrotic areas may considerably improve symptoms and quality of life. However, it has not been established whether the reduction of tumor mass by surgical intervention improves outcome [6]. Determining the tumor extent (localization and metastases) as well as the primary tumor location is an essential aspect of the management of endocrine tumors, because it is a basic condition for resection. Certain locations, such as the small bowel, can be associated with multicentricity, and care should be taken to ensure adequate resection.

With the preoperative injection of radiolabelled somatostatin analogues, it is possible to identify endocrine tumors intraoperatively and to determine the extent of disease without extensive dissection. Therefore, external scintigraphy combined with intraoperative gamma emission detection might be used to decrease the high rate of unsuccessful surgical explorations. It should be noted that in some series the negative laparotomy rate for patients with pancreatic and ileal endocrine tumors has been reported to be as high as 30%.

Pancreatic Endocrine Tumors

Pancreatic endocrine tumors are difficult to localize. The most common functional endocrine pancreatic tumor is insulinoma. Those arising sporadically are generally solitary lesions, although seemingly sporadic cases with multiple tumors have been reported. These tumors are almost exclusively confined to the pancreas, but they may arise in aberrant pancreatic tissue. Gastrinoma is frequently a duodenal tumor. As many as 40% of gastrinomas may occur in the setting of MEN-1. Unlike insulinomas, most sporadic gastrinomas are malignant. They metastasize to regional lymph nodes and the liver, and less commonly to distant sites. Sporadic gastrinomas are usually solitary and vary in size from sub-centimetric lesions to >3 cm in diameter. Most of these tumors are located in the gastrinoma triangle (defined by the confluence of the cystic and common hepatic ducts, the border of the second and third portions of the duodenum, and the neck of the pancreas) but ectopic locations such as the jejunum, stomach, mesentery, spleen, and ovaries have been reported. Surgical exploration is recommended for all sporadic cases of gastrinoma without evidence of hepatic metastasis [7]. Endosonography is highly accurate in the localization of gastric and pancreatic neuroendocrine tumors and is cost effective when used early in the preoperative localization strategy. Up to 20% of insulinomas are not palpable at the time of surgery, whereas gastrinomas are not found during surgery in up to 40% of cases. Concerning the intraoperative tumor localization rate, the combination of intraoperative ultrasound and surgical palpation leads to 97% cure rate in patients with benign insulinomas. Furthermore, intraoperative ultrasound does not allow accurate detection of small lymph node metastases because of their normal size. Therefore, the intraoperative use of gamma probes makes it possible to identify recurrent tumor tissue when the normal anatomy has been altered or primary tumors in unusual anatomic locations. Unfortunately, there is no published experience apart from some heterogeneous case reports.

Carcinoid Tumors of the Small Intestine

Small intestinal carcinoids may be multiple: 87% occur within the ileum, and 40% present within 2 feet of the ileocaecal valve [6]. Primary tumors tend to remain small, and sometimes a metastasis in the liver is the first clinical appearance of a non-functioning tumor. In patients with midgut carcinoids, 123I-MIBG tumor uptake is found with a sensitivity of 40% to 68%, whereas only 37% of foregut carcinoids can be localized. Somatostatin receptor scintigraphy is currently the investigation of choice for the staging and identification of the primary carcinoid lesion. This functional imaging modality has an 83% diagnostic accuracy and a positive predictive value of 100%, and can also identify lesions not viewed by radiological methods [8]. CT and MRI are less sensitive than radionuclide imaging using 111In-octreotide, because they identify only approximately 50% of the primary tumors. The combined SPECT-CT device provides both functional and anatomical information; it affected the diagnostic interpretation of somatostatin receptor scintigraphy in 32% of the patients with neuroendocrine tumors and led to alterations in the therapeutic strategy in 14% of patients. Radioguided surgery may be helpful in detecting multicentric disease and in checking residual disease to obtain complete tumor ablation; however, at present no prospective studies are available.

Colonic and Rectal Carcinoid Tumors

Colonic carcinoid tumors are rare, and are seldom multicentric. They occur more often in the right part of the colon. Patients with colonic carcinoid tumors usually have non-specific symptoms and present at a later stage than those with small bowel or appendiceal carcinoid tumors. Most patients require colonic resection with locoregional lymphadenectomy. Intraoperative gamma probe detection is not of particular interest in this setting. Rectal carcinoid tumors are usually of hindgut origin and rarely secrete serotonin. Approximately half of the patients with rectal carcinoid tumors present with rectal bleeding, pain, or constipation, whereas the other half are asymptomatic and are diagnosed during screening colonoscopy. Metastatic disease is rare in lesions smaller than 1 cm, but common in those larger than 2 cm [9]. Small lesions are managed with local excision or endoscopic resection, whereas larger (>2 cm) ones or those that invade the muscularis mucosa are usually treated by a low anterior resection or abdominoperineal resection. [123I-Tyr3] and 111In-labeled somatostatin analogues have been successfully used for intraoperative detection of neuroendocrine tumors. Radioguided surgery identified 57% more gastroenteropancreatic tumors when compared to the "palpating finger" of the surgeon. Preoperative receptor imaging is particularly efficient for tumors larger than 10 mm, with a detection rate of 92%, in contrast to 38% for gastroenteropancreatic tumors less than 10 mm in size. Use of an intraoperative gamma probe revealed abdominal small endocrine tumor sites accumulating (111In- DTPA-D-Phe1)-pentetreotide more efficiently (>90% of all tumors investigated) than somatostatin receptor scintigraphy (68 to 77%), because lesions of more than 5 mm in size could be identified. Tracers such as

68Ga-DOTA-NOC or 64Cu-TETAoctreotide seem to be of the greatest clinical interest for radioguided surgery, because they exhibit better tumor-to-background ratios than 111In-octreotide and have demonstrated significantly more lesions in patients with neuroendocrine tumors [10].

Radioguided Surgery: The Sentinel Node Concept

Melanoma

Sentinel lymph node biopsy is accepted worldwide as the method of choice to stage regional lymph nodes in patients with melanoma, even at unexpected/abnormal draining sites (which have a frequency of about 5%). Because there are often many nodes (radioactive and/or coloured), it is difficult to establish which are the true sentinel lymph nodes. In the Sunbelt Melanoma Trial of 1,184 patients, it was found that sometimes the most radioactive lymph node was negative for metastatic involvement, whereas other, less radioactive lymph nodes were metastatic (13.1% of cases) [11]. It appears reasonable therefore to recommend resection and histological analysis of all "blue" nodes and nodes with radioactivity count rates greater than 10% of the ex vivo count rate of the node with the greatest radioactivity. This approach should reduce the risk of false-negative biopsies. Another issue concerns the reliability of the histological analysis of the node. A consensus is emerging that frozen section and H&E staining alone have too low a sensitivity for clinical use, since they demonstrate metastasis in less than 50% of the lymph nodes that actually harbor melanoma cells [12]. Additional analysis with step sections and immunohistochemical staining increases the sensitivity. Radioguided surgery is particularly useful in patients with melanomas that are located in the perineum, since lymph drainage is clinically ambiguous. These lesions may drain to nodes in the groin, iliac, and obturator regions, as demonstrated by lymphoscintigraphy. Regional lymph node metastases (N1 to N3) define stage III disease and are cardinal prognostic variables for patients with cutaneous melanoma. Since patients with melanomas <1 mm thick rarely have nodal disease, sentinel node biopsy is not commonly performed in this group, but should be considered when negative prognostic features such as ulceration or Clark level IV to V invasion are present. For patients with melanomas that are >1 mm thick, sentinel node staging can be considered for prognostic purposes, and to evaluate eligibility for clinical trials and the need for adjuvant therapy. Accurate staging can identify patients whose risk of recurrence is sufficiently high to justify adjuvant systemic treatment.

Breast

Staging of the axilla can be based on either axillary dissection or sentinel lymph node biopsy. In the first instance, resection of the first level lymph nodes (lower axilla) is required for histopathological classification. The specimen usually contains six or more lymph nodes; if less than six nodes are examined and they are negative for metastatic involvement, the classification is pN0. In the case of sentinel lymph node biopsy, if only the sentinel node is resected and examined (without total axillary dissection), this factor is reported with a specific notation, for example pN1(sn). Although some investigators have reservations about this approach, the revised TNM classification recognizes that sentinel lymph node biopsy (including both lymphoscintigraphic mapping and intraoperative gamma probe detection) plays an important role in the care of patients with breast cancer. Nevertheless, consideration should be paid to some limiting factors of the procedure, such as partial lymphatic drainage to the internal mammary chain (in about 17% of the cases, if the radiocolloid is injected peritumorally), depending on the location of the primary tumor within the breast [13]. It is unclear whether lymphatic mapping and sentinel lymph node biopsy should be performed in patients with ductal carcinoma in situ. By definition, an in-situ breast cancer should not yet have invaded the lymphatic channels, yet foci of microinfiltration can be observed at extensive histopathology of some resected cancers that had been defined as in situ before resection [14]. Another issue concerns the possibility of predicting metastases in non-sentinel nodes, when the sentinel lymph node is positive for metastasis (an event reported to occur in about 50% of cases). A confounding variable in patients treated with neoadjuvant chemotherapy before surgery is fibrosis of the lymphatic channels, which can raise the rate of false-negative sentinel lymph node biopsies in up to 33% of cases [15]. It is generally agreed that the combined use of a dye and radiotracer yields better identification rates. The intraoperative analysis of the excised sentinel lymph node using "touch imprints" is fast, convenient, and highly sensitive for detecting tumor cells in the lymph node. On the other hand, staging of a residual tumor (R0, R1, R2) is not influenced if a marginal, apical, or sentinel node is metastatic.

Head and Neck Cancers

The usefulness of sentinel lymph node biopsy in tumors of the thyroid, salivary glands, or squamous cell cancers of the head and neck is still not established. It is clear that lymphoscintigraphic mapping identifies bilateral draining basins, suggesting nodal sites that can be sampled for staging, leading to selective nodal dissection or conservative management [16]. In the neck, there are about 200 lymph nodes, with many separate anatomic structures adjacent to one another, so often the primary tumor and draining lymph nodes are in close proximity. On the other hand, elective neck dissection reveals lymph node metastases in an average 30% of clinically N0 patients, so in about 70% of patients this operation is unnecessary. Even the most advanced nuclear medicine imaging method, positron emission tomography (PET, which is useful for detecting local recurrences), is largely ineffective for evaluating tumor status of the sentinel lymph node(s), as well as of the second-echelon and contralateral nodes. Therefore, lymphoscintigraphic mapping holds promise for guiding surgery, although larger trials and further experience (with longer follow-up studies) are necessary before radioguided sentinel lymph node biopsy becomes the standard of care for planning treatment [17]. Different figures have been reported for clinically occult metastatic involvement of sentinel lymph node(s) identified under radioguidance: 21% of oropharyngeal cancer, 34% of squamous cell cancers of the tongue, and 34% and 45% respectively of oral and tongue cancers. However, in a series of 41 patients with primary head and neck cancers, radioguided sentinel lymph node identification failed in 3/9 patients with metastatic lymph nodes [18]. Sentinel node biopsy can modify the prognostic assessment and is helpful for selecting patients for adjuvant therapies and/or more aggressive treatment protocols. In contrast to melanoma, here intraoperative frozen-section histopathology seems to be more reliable, since only 4 of 48 patients with metastatic involvement of the sentinel lymph node were missed on frozen-section analysis.

Gastrointestinal Tract

Both blue dye and radiocolloids are used for lymph node mapping and identification of the sentinel node in patients with cancer of the gastrointestinal tract. Interstitial injection is performed either submucosally around the tumor (during endoscopy prior to surgery) or subserosally (during open or laparoscopic surgery) [19].

In esophageal cancer, a close correlation has been found between the number of sentinel lymph nodes (identified with the use of 99mTc-labeled rhenium sulphide), lymph node status, pathological stage, and the number of metastatic nodes. Sentinel lymph node biopsy is especially useful in minimally invasive surgery. Lymph nodal status is the most powerful prognostic factor in esophageal cancer, and accurate staging is necessary to distinguish potentially curable patients from those with local advanced disease. Although esophagectomy remains the standard of care in early-stage tumors (stage I, IIA), its role is being questioned in patients with locally advanced disease (stage IIB, III) because of the generally poor outcomes following surgical resection alone. The overall 5-year survival rate for patients with esophageal cancer is 20% to 25% (60% to 70% for patients with stage I disease, 5% to 10% for patients with stage III disease).

In Japan, the high incidence of gastric cancer has led to the evaluation of sentinel lymph node biopsy for patients with this type of tumor. The standard treatment for early cases is gastrectomy with en bloc lymph node dissection. Lymphatic mapping has disclosed unexpected/aberrant sites of drainage, thus guiding surgeons to perform a regional dissection approach tailored to the individual patient. Both conventional histochemistry and molecular biology techniques have been applied in the search for micrometastatic involvement of the sentinel lymph node(s) [19].

Multiple reports exist in the literature on the feasibility of radioguided SLN biopsy for gastric cancer [20]. Many of these reports from eastern Asia specifically target a purely laparoscopic approach to radioguided SLN biopsy in the treatment of cases of early stage gastric cancer [21]. Most frequently, 99mTc tin colloid has been used as the radiocolloid, especially in eastern Asia. However, 99mTc colloidal rhenium sulphide, 99mTc sulphur colloid and 99mTc colloidal human albumin have also been utilized. These radiocolloid agents are generally injected endoscopically in up to four submucosal sites around the tumor in a period from two to 24 hours before surgery. The two largest series reported are by Kitagawa et al. [22] and Uenosono et al. [23]. In 2002, Kitagawa et al. [22] identified an SLN in 138 of 145 patients (95.2%) with presumed cT1N0 or cT2N0 gastric cancer. An SLN was positive in 22 of 24 patients who had lymph node metastases and this demonstrated a diagnostic accuracy of assessment of the regional lymph node status on the basis of the SLN status of 98.6%. In 2005, Uenosono et al. [23] identified an SLN in 99 of 104 patients (95.2%) with presumed cT1 or cT2 gastric cancer. Excluding three technical failures in radiocolloid injection, identification rates were 99% (78 of 79) and 95% (21 of 22) for cT1 and cT2 lesions, respectively. Lymph node metastases and/or micrometastases were found in 28 patients (15 cT1 and 13 cT2) and the resultant false-negative rate, sensitivity, and accuracy were significantly better for cT1 tumors than for cT2 tumors ($p<0.001$, $p=0.004$, and $p<0.001$, respectively). While the possibility exists for radioguided SLN biopsy to help individualize the surgical therapy for patients with early stage gastric cancer, additional studies are needed to determine its utility.

Aberrant lymph drainage leading to modification of the intended surgical approach can be identified as well in 5% to 8% of patients with colorectal cancer. Lymphatic mapping and sentinel lymph node analysis performed with molecular biology techniques can detect micrometastases in up to 14% of the cases, identifying a subgroup of patients who can benefit from adjuvant chemotherapy. In a study of 492 consecutive patients (401 with colon cancer, 91 with rectal cancer), the overall success rate for radioguided sentinel lymph node identification was 97.8%, with most of the failures occurring in rectal cancers (8.8% of the cases, versus 0.7% for colon cancer), most likely due to local submucosal lymphatic fibrosis induced by neoadjuvant radiation therapy administered prior to surgery [24]. The overall accuracy rate for predicting lymph node metastases was 95.4% (with 89.3% sensitivity), while the overall incidence of skip metastasis was 10.9%. A minimum number of lymph nodes must be assessed for accurate staging of patients with colorectal cancer, as nodal status (the number of nodes resected and the presence of micrometastases) is crucial for planning treatment after primary surgery. Inadequate retrieval and assessment of sentinel lymph nodes is associated with worse outcome (e.g., in stage II patients) [25]. Although lymph node mapping per se (either with blue dye or radiocolloids) does not generally modify the surgical procedure (which usually follows a standardized approach), it does identify the crucial node(s) to be submitted to extensive analysis with sophisticated laboratory techniques searching for micrometastases. Adjuvant chemotherapy is performed in the positive cases. The lymphotropic agents are most frequently injected subserosally during open surgery, with a specificity approaching 100% when using the blue dye, and during laparoscopic procedures [25]. Submucosal injection is generally performed during endoscopy prior to surgery, and the use of radiocolloids is increasing. The potential advantages of lymphatic mapping for patients with colorectal cancers and malignant polyps are less obvious than for those with breast cancer or melanoma, and the procedure is generally performed in strictly controlled clinical trials.

Anal cancer

Anal cancer is a rare disease, accounting for approximately 1.85% of digestive system cancers. In the USA, an estimated 5,070 new cases (2,020 men and 3,050 women) of anal cancer (involving the anus, anal canal, or anorectum) and 680 deaths from the disease were expected to occur in 2008. Human papilloma virus infection, cervical dysplasia or cancer, HIV seropositivity, low CD4 count, cigarette smoking, anoreceptive intercourse, and immunosuppression following solid organ transplant are known risk factors for anal cancer. Before the mid-1980s, the treatment of choice for anal cancer was abdominoperineal resection (APR). The 5-year survival rate after APR for anal cancer was 40–70%, with worse outcomes for patients with larger tumors and nodal metastases. In the 1920s and 1930s, inguinal node dissection was included in the surgical management of these patients, although it was generally reserved for those with clinically enlarged (although not necessarily involved) inguinal nodes. By the 1950s, it had became clear that the morbidity associated with lymph node dissection was much greater than any survival benefit, and the procedure was gradually abandoned. In 1974, Nigro et al. [26] proposed a multimodality approach to treatment, combining radiation and chemotherapy, which has since become the standard treatment. Local control rates of 60–90% over all stages are achievable, with sphincter preservation in approximately 65% of patients. The prognosis after combined radiochemotherapy for anal cancer may be influenced by several factors: high tumor stage and regional nodal involvement, tumor site in the anal canal, and inguinal lymph node involvement in anal canal carcinoma. Synchronous inguinal metastases have been reported in 10–25% of patients and metachronous metastases in 5–25% [27]. An array of tools for assessing inguinal metastasis has been proposed, including clinical examination, endosonography, computed tomography (CT), and magnetic resonance imaging (MRI); however, they are unable to detect nodal involvement in all cases. Furthermore, only histological studies can confirm metastasis in an enlarged node or a micrometastasis in a normal-sized node. In recent years, sentinel node biopsy (SNB) has proven to be a safe and effective technique for sampling inguinal sentinel lymph nodes [28,29]. Since 2001, SNB in patients with anal cancer has improved the accuracy of inguinal staging and the planning of radiotherapy treatment, obviating the need for inguinal radiotherapy and eliminating its related morbidity in patients without metastasis at SLN biopsy. In their recent review of the literature, Damin et al. [28] evaluated 84 patients by SLN sampling: the detection rate was between 66 and 100%, and metastases were found in 7.1–42.0% of the patients. No major complications were reported. Gretschel et al. [30] subsequently described their experience with 40 patients. In contrast to their previous reports, the rate of anal cancer detection was 56% in inguinal lymph nodes (76% in a previous series), and 30% in inguinal node metastases (42% previously). The authors suggested that SLN biopsy in anal cancer can be used to appropriately select patients for inguinal irradiation, especially those with T1 and T2 tumors. These patients receive either additional treatment or are spared unnecessary radiation. SLN biopsy is not currently recommended for larger (T3/T4) tumors or in patients with prior surgical manipulation of the anal or inguinal region. Mistrangelo et al., in a study of 43 patients with anal cancer, used a radioguided technique [31], which yielded a detection rate of 97.7% in inguinal lymph nodes, with 18.6% of inguinal node metastases (42% previously).

Urogenital and Gynaecological Cancers

In cancers of the prostate preoperatively staged as N0, the optimal extent of regional lymph node dissection is under debate. Preliminary reports indicate that in prostate cancer, the extent of lymph node dissection might be guided by the metastatic status of the sentinel lymph node, especially if it is found in unexpected, extraregional locations [32]. For penile cancer (a typical tumor of the midline, in which bilateral lymphatic drainage is the rule) sentinel lymph node biopsy may spare unnecessary bilateral (heavy) groin lymph node dissection, a surgical procedure with a heavy burden of morbidity and side effects, and at the same time result in considerable improvement in quality of life [33]. Interesting studies have been published on sentinel lymph node biopsy in patients with vulvar or cervical cancers [34,35], where lymphatic mapping is performed with blue dye and/or radiocolloids during either open or laparoscopic surgery. The success rate in sentinel lymph node identification is generally high, and the status of the node plays an important role in the selection of more or less aggressive therapeutic approaches. Regional lymph node status is a major prognostic factor for the therapeutic strategy of gynaecological malignancies. Early cervical cancer is treated with surgery and/or radiotherapy; surgery consists of radical hysterectomy and pelvic lymphadenectomy. However, metastasis in pelvic lymph nodes is found in only 15% of the women with stage Ib cervical cancer [36] and thus the vast majority of these patients do not benefit from surgical treatment associated with considerable morbidity (nerve and vessel damage, lymphedema). As in other applications of surgical oncology, sentinel lymph node biopsy could represent a definite advantage to select women for whom lymphadenectomy is really necessary. Similar considerations also apply to patients with vulvar cancer, a condition in which the status of the regional lymph nodes is crucial for therapeutic decision making. Standard treatment includes bilateral inguinofemoral lymphadenectomy, but this surgery is associated with high rates of short-term and long-term morbidity, and only 10% to 26% of patients with vulvar cancer have inguinal metastases. Therefore, the majority of early-stage patients unnecessarily undergo overtreatment (i.e., lymphadenectomy with an ensuing negative impact on quality of life). Sentinel lymph node biopsy could ensure accurate lymph node staging as a prerequisite to implementing less aggressive treatments, especially in patients with early vulvar cancer.

New Perspectives: Preferential Migration of Activated NK Cells to Tumor Tissues as a Tool to Radioguided Surgery

NK cells are the effectors of native (as opposed to adaptive) anti-tumor cytotoxicity [37]. They exert their anti-tumoral activity mainly through serine esterase (perforin and granzyme) mediated cell cytotoxicity. At least in resting NK cells, the only activating receptor inducing efficient cytotoxicity appears to be CD16. CD16 engagement by its ligand, IgG Fc, triggers degranulation [38]. Another marker of NK cells is CD56. Most blood NK cells display the (CD56^{low} CD16+) phenotype, only a minority being (CD56^{high} CD16-). In activated NK cells the responsiveness of the natural cytotoxicity receptors is strongly upregulated. In particular, activation by IL-2 promotes LAK activity by inducing perforin- and granzyme-dependent lysis of target cells. These properties of NK cells have opened up the possibility of NK cell-based immunotherapy against some malignancies [39].

A critical issue in therapy of metastatic disease is the optimization of NK cell migration to tumor tissues and their persistence therein. NK are rapidly recruited from the blood into injured tissues during inflammation, viral infection and tumor growth. NK cell recruitment is governed by integrated signals, which include adhesion molecules and chemotactic factors. CD56^{low} CD16^{+} NK cells express both β1 and β2 integrins, as well as the ligands for E- and P-selectins. The mechanism of NK cell recruitment appears to involve chemokines such as CXCL8, CCL3 and CX3CL1. Indeed most classical NK cells (CD56^{low} CD16^{+}) express CXCR1 and CX3CR1 while the minor CD56^{high} CD16-NK subset express CCR7 [40]. On the basis of their surface phenotype it is conceivable that CD56^{low} CD16^{+} cells may be mainly recruited in pathogen-invaded inflamed tissues, whereas CD56^{high} CD16-cells may be essentially attracted by secondary lymphoid compartments such as lymph nodes.

Indirect evidence for NK cell targeting of human tumor comes from observations of NK cell infiltration in some solid tumors [41]. The ability of NK cells to migrate to tumor sites appears to be tightly linked to their stage of activation. Limited numbers (<300 mm^{-2} tumor tissue) of NK cells were found in pulmonary B16 melanoma metastases. However, within 16 h of treatment with IL-2, there was a significant rise (1.5-fold) in the number of intra-tumoral NK cells, and at 48 h the number had increased 4- to 5-fold compared with non-treated animals. Therefore, although the number of NK cells in malignant tissues is usually small, systemic treatment with IL-2 together with adoptive transfer of mitogen-stimulated, lymphokine-activated T killer (T-LAK) increased accumulation of these cells in tumors. The relevance of the route of administration on tumor localization was explored on a B16 melanoma metastatic model [42]. T-LAK cells were labelled with ^{125}I-dU or the fluorescent dye tetramethylrhodamine isothiocyanate (TRITC) and transferred by intravenous-cardiac, intravenous-portal or intravenous-peritoneal injection. Intravenously injected T-LAK were mainly found in lung metastases. Following locoregional administration of T-LAK cells into the portal vein, tenfold higher numbers (from 30 to 400 cells/mm^{2}) were found in hepatic metastases than were observed following intravenous or intracardiac injection. In the liver, a surprisingly large number of intraportally injected T-LAK cells (approx. 1300/mm^{2}) were observed to accumulate in the perivascular spaces of the portal, but not the central veins. Therefore, T-LAK cells are able to localize substantially into tumor metastases in various anatomical locations, but mainly following locoregional injection.

Due to their tumor infiltrating capability, adoptive transfer of A-NK has recently been exploited as a method for targeting products of genes to tumor site. IL-12 transduced A-NK cells localized 10- to 50-fold better within lung metastases than in the surrounding normal lung tissue [43].

Migration of A-NK to Hepatic Metastasis and Imaging Studies

Hepatic metastatic carcinoma is a clinical indication where NK cell function likely impacts the progression of disease. The liver is the most common site of metastasis in patients with colorectal cancer (CRC) and is a common site of metastasis for other gastrointestinal malignancies, such as pancreatic cancer. Liver metastases are solely fed by the hepatic artery, and injection of chemotherapeutic agents via this route has proven to be effective in controlling the spread of tumors of the digestive tract. Intrahepatic administration of A-NK in a syngeneic rat liver metastasis model, the CC531 colon carcinoma cell line, was used to study the homing properties and anti-tumor effects of adoptively transferred, interleukin-2 (IL-2)-activated, cultured natural killer (A-NK) [44]. The routes chosen in that study were: jugular vein, portal vein, hepatic artery and the peritoneal cavity (i.p). The rats were sacrificed 20 h after administration of A-NK cells. The highest ($p<0.05$) infiltration of tumors by A-NK cells was found both at the tumor border and in the tumor centre after injection via the hepatic artery.

Although injection of A-NK cells into the hepatic artery may be an ideal approach to treating tumors metastasizing to the liver, no evidence exists in humans for the superior tumor homing of locoregional vs. systemic A-NK delivery. In a recent study we showed that A-NK injected A-NK cells adoptively transferred to the liver via the intra-arterial route have preferential access to and substantial accumulation at the tumor site [45]. Adherent NK (A-NK) cells employed in our study constitute a subset of IL-2-stimulated NK cells which show increased expression of integrins and the ability to adhere to solid surface and to migrate, infiltrate, and destroy cancer. Five hundred million A-NK cells with a donor-dependent CD56[+]CD16[+]CD3[−] (NK) or CD56[+]CD16[+]CD3[+] (NKT) phenotype were obtained from a 160 mL sample after fifteen days of culture with IL-2. A-NK cells labelled with ^{111}In-oxine were injected intra-arterially in the liver of three colon carcinoma patients with liver metastases. For delivery of A-NK cells, the hepatic arterial catheter implanted for chemotherapeutical purposes was used. After 30 days, each patient had a new preparation of ^{111}In-A-NK cells injected intravenously. Migration of these cells to various organs was evaluated by Planar whole-body and single-photon emission-computed tomography (SPECT) and their differential localization to non-pathological liver parenchyma and tumor lesions was assessed by intravenous injection of ^{99m}Tc-phytate. When injected intravenously, these cells localized to the lung before being visible in the spleen and liver. In contrast, localization of intra-arterially injected A-NK cells was virtually confined to the spleen and liver. Importantly, binding of A-NK cells to liver neoplastic tissues was observed only after intra-arterial injections.

This model has allowed us to formally define the preferential migratory capacity of activated NK cells to the tumor in vivo and to compare for the first time in the same patient the relative efficiency of different routes of cell delivery. The possibility of obtaining large numbers of tumor-homing autologous lymphocytes from low blood volumes may extend their application to multiple diagnostic approaches: i.e., pre-surgical injection of labelled A-NK cells could allow intra-surgical detection and removal of liver micrometases.

Future Perspectives

Target-cell contact is preceded by extensive cytokinetic manoeuvres by NK cells through microvessel walls and basal lamina, and through the extracellular space. Tridimensional culture will help understand the application of A-NK tumor migration to the highly demanding application of radioguided surgery.

References

1. Povoski S, Neff RL, Mojzisik CM et al (2009) A comprehensive overview of radioguided surgery using gamma detection probe technology. World J Surg Oncol 7:11
2. Rampaul RS, Bagnall M, Burrell H et al (2004) Randomized clinical trial comparing radioisotope occult lesion localization and wire-guided excision for biopsy of occult breast lesions. Br J Surg 91:1575–1577
3. Ronka R, Krogerus L, Leppanen E et al (2004) Radio-guided occult lesion localization in patients undergoing breast conserving surgery and sentinel node biopsy. Am J Surg 187:491–496
4. Norman J (2004) Minimally invasive parathyroid surgery. Recent trends becoming standard of care yielding smaller, more successful operations at a lower cost. Otolaryngol Clin North Am 37:683–688
5. Mariani G, Gulec SA, Rubello D et al (2003) Preoperative localisation and radioguided parathyroid surgery. J Nucl Med 44:1443–1458
6. Modlin IM, Lye KD, Kidd M (2003) A 5-decade analysis of 13,715 carcinoid tumors. Cancer 97:934–959
7. Viola KV, Sosa JA (2005) Current advances in the diagnosis and treatment of pancreatic endocrine tumors. Curr Opin Oncol 17:24–27
8. Ricke J, Klose KJ, Mignon M et al (2001) Standardization of imaging in neuroendocrine tumors: results of a European Delphi process. Eur J Radiol 37:8–17
9. Soga J (1997) Carcinoids of the rectum: an evaluation of 1271 reported cases. Surg Today 27:112–119
10. Anderson CJ, Dehdashti F, Cutler PD et al (2001) 64Cu-TETAoctreotide as a PET imaging agent for patients with neuroendocrine tumors. J Nucl Med 42:213–221
11. Ribuffo D, Gradilone A, Vonella M et al (2003) Prognostic significance of reverse transcriptase-polymerase chain reaction-negative sentinel nodes in malignant melanoma. Ann Surg Oncol 10:396–402
12. Gershenwald JE, Uren RF, Mariani G, Thompson JF (2006) Sentinel lymph node biopsy in cutaneous melanoma. In: Mariani G, Giuliano AE, Strauss HW (eds) Radioguided surgery: a comprehensive team approach. Springer, New York pp 98–116
13. Cody HS (2002) Sentinel lymph node biopsy. London: Martin Dunitz, pp 177–275
14. Wilke LG, McCall LM, Posther KE et al (2006) Surgical complications associated with sentinel lymph node biopsy: results from a prospective international cooperative group trial. Ann

Surg Oncol 13:491–500

15. Obenaus E, Erba PA, Chinol M et al (2006) Radiopharmaceuticals for radioguided surgery. In: Mariani G, Giuliano AE, Strauss HW (eds) Radioguided surgery: a comprehensive team approach. Springer, New York pp 3–11

16. Stoeckli SJ, Pfaltz M, Ross G et al (2005) The second international conference on sentinel node biopsy in mucosal head and neck cancer. Ann Surg Oncol 12:919–924

17. Ross GL, Soutar DS, MacDonald G et al (2004) Sentinel node biopsy in head and neck cancer: preliminary results of a multi-center trial. Ann Surg Oncol 11:690–696

18. De Cicco C, Trifirò G, Calabrese L et al (2006) Lymphatic mapping to tailor selective lymphadenectomy in tongue carcinoma cN0: beyond the sentinel node concept. Eur J Nucl Med Mol Imaging 33:900–905

19. Kitagawa Y, Fujii H, Mukai M et al (2005) Sentinel lymph node mapping in esophageal and gastric cancer–impact on individualized minimally invasive surgery. In: Leong S, Kitajima M, Kitagawa Y (eds) Selective sentinel lymphadenectomy for human solid cancer. New York, Springer Science, pp 123–139

20. Gretschel S, Bembenek A, Hünerbein M et al (2007) Efficacy of different technical procedures for sentinel lymph node biopsy in gastric cancer staging. Ann Surg Oncol 14:2028–2035

21. Saikawa Y, Otani Y, Kitagawa Y et al (2006) Interim results of sentinel node biopsy during laparoscopic gastrectomy: possible role in function-preserving surgery for early cancer. World J Surg 30:1962–1968

22. Kitagawa Y, Fujii H, Mukai M et al (2002) Radioguided sentinel node detection for gastric cancer. Br J Surg 89:604–608

23. Uenosono Y, Natsugoe S, Ehi K et al (2005) Detection of sentinel nodes and micrometastases using radioisotope navigation and immunohistochemistry in patients with gastric cancer. Br J Surg 92:886–889

24. Bilchik A, Saha S, Tsioulias G et al (2001) Aberrant drainage of missed micrometastases: the value of lymphatic mapping and focused analysis of sentinel lymph nodes in gastrointestinal neoplasms. Ann Surg Oncol 8:82–85

25. Saha S, Dan AG, Viehl CT et al (2005) Sentinel lymph node mapping in colon and rectal cancer–its impact on staging, limitations, and pitfalls. In: Leong S, Kitajima M, Kitagawa Y (eds) Selective sentinel lymphadenectomy for human solid cancer. New York, Springer Science

26. Nigro ND, Vaitkeicus VK, Basil B (1974) Combined therapy for cancer of the anal canal: A preliminary report. Dis Colon Rectum 17:354–356

27. Gerard J-P, Chapet O, Samiei F et al (2001) Management of inguinal lymph node metastases in patients with carcinoma of the anal canal. Experience in a series of 270 patients treated in Lyon and review of the literature. Cancer 92:77–84

28. Damin DC, Rosito MA, Schwartsmann G (2006) Sentinel lymph node in carcinoma of the anal canal: A review. EJSO 32:247–252

29 Mistrangelo M, Bello` M, Mobiglia A et al (2009) Feasibility of the sentinel node biopsy in anal cancer. Q J Nucl Med Mol Imaging 53:3–8

30. Gretschel S, Warnick P, Bembenek A et al (2008). Lymphatic mapping and sentinel lymph node biopsy in epidermoid carcinoma of the anal canal. Eur J Surg Oncol 34:890–894.

31. Mistrangelo M, Morino M (2009) Sentinel lymph node biopsy in anal cancer: a review Gastroeneterol clin biol 33:446-450

32. Takashima H, Egawa M, Imao T et al (2004) Validity of sentinel lymph node concept for patients with prostate cancer. J Urol 71:2268–2271

33. Kroon BK, Horenblas S, Meinhardt W et al (2005) Dynamic sentinel node biopsy in penile carcinoma: evaluation of 10 years experience. Eur Urol 47:601–606

34. Merisio C, Berretta R, Gualdi M et al (2005) Radioguided sentinel lymph node detection in vulvar cancer. Int J Gynecol Cancer 15:493–497

35. Barranger E, Grahek D, Cortez A et al (2003) Laparoscopic sentinel lymph node procedure

using a combination of patent blue and radioisotope in women with cervical carcinoma. Cancer 97:3003–3009

36. Lantzsch T, Wolters M, Grimm J et al (2001) Sentinel node procedure in Ib cervical cancer: a preliminary series. Br J Cancer 14:791–794

37. Waldhauer I, Steile A (2008) NK cells and cancer immunosurveillance. Oncogene 45:5932–5943

38. Bryceson YT, March ME, Ljunggren HG et al (2006) Synergy among receptors on resting NK cells for the activation of natural cytotoxicity and cytokine secretion. Blood 107:159–166

39. Terme M, Ullrich E, Delahaye NF et al (2008) Natural killer cell-directed therapies: moving from unexpected results to successful strategies. Nat Immunol 9:486–494

40. Cooper MA, Fehniger TA, Caligiuri MA (2001) The biology of human natural killer-cell subsets. Trends Immunol 22:633–640

41. Albertsson PA, Basse PH, Hokland M et al (2003) NK cells and the tumor microenvironment: implications for NK-cell function and anti-tumor activity. Trends Immunol 24:603–609

42. Kjaergaard J, Hokland ME, Agger R et al (2000) Biodistribution and tumor localization of lymphokine-activated killer T cells following different routes of administration into tumor-bearing animals. Cancer Immunol Immunother 48:550–560

43. Goding S, Yang Q, Mi Z et al (2007) Targeting of products of genes to tumor sites using adoptively transferred A-NK and T-LAK cells. Cancer Gene Ther 14:441–450

44. Hagenaars M, Ensink NG, Koelemij R et al (1998) Regional administration of natural killer cells in a rat hepatic metastasis model results in better tumor infiltration and anti-tumor response than systemic administration. Int J Cancer 75:233–238

45. Matera L, Galetto A, Bello M et al (2006) In vivo migration of labeled autologous natural killer cells to liver metastases in patients with colon carcinoma. J Transl Med 14:4–49

Prosthetic Materials in Surgical Oncology

4

F. Trombetta, T. Lubrano

The use of prostheses in surgery is nowadays widespread, though some doubts still remain on the hypothetical carcinogenicity of these prostheses. Some investigational trials have shown the possibility of carcinogenic stimulation by foreign bodies introduced into the body, like those by Vasiliev and Moizhess in 1982 [1], where polyvinyl hydrochloride film was inserted into the abdomen of some rats and some sarcomatous cells were subsequently introduced. It was then possible to observe an increase in the rate and decrease in growth times of sarcomas thus induced.

The mechanism of this effect was suggested in 1975 by Brand et al. [2], who asserted that the reaction of a foreign body creates the conditions required for the neoplastic development and maturation of cells with a neoplastic determination already present in the body, although without inducing their mutation in itself.

Some cases have been reported in the literature of angiosarcomas and sarcomas of other origin associated with stimulation by a foreign body as referred by Jennings et al. [3]. The authors affirmed that the introduction of a foreign body should however be considered a factor able to induce the onset of sarcomas.

In contrast, more recently in 2002 Ghadimi et al. [4] showed in a molecular study that although millions of hernia repairs are performed in the world with prostheses, no patient has subsequently reported the development of a soft tissue tumor. The analysis of proliferation markers and apoptosis, as well as the modulation of hot shock proteins, do not seem to prove the carcinogenic potential of prosthetic materials.

However, there are no studies in the literature regarding the implant of tumor cells on mesh, following reparative surgery in oncological patients. The incorporating mechanisms of the prostheses and their rehabilitation on neoformed tissues in the case of biological prostheses could favor the intraperitoneal implant of neoplastic cells, even though there have only been reports of isolated cases, such as the

F. Trombetta (✉)
Surgical Oncology Unit, S. Giovanni Battista University Hospital, Turin, Italy

New Technologies in Surgical Oncology. Antonio Mussa (Ed.)
© Springer-Verlag Italia 2010

onset of peritoneal metastases on the prosthesis of a plug-and-mesh repair in a patient with advanced gastric tumor [5]. Definitive proof, however, does not exist and no randomized trial has ever been conducted, so such case reports cannot be considered elements against the use of this mesh.

In the light of these data, therefore, the use of prostheses in oncological surgery has been constantly increasing, permitting extreme situations to be resolved and enabling more radical surgery, with the possibilities of reconstruction being considerably increased by the availability of more and more innovative aids.

The oncological surgery fields where prostheses are now largely used can be singled out as:
1. Oncological surgery in the true sense
2. Surgery for wall defects
3. Surgery for inguinal hernia.

Oncological Surgery in the True Sense

Modern oncological surgery makes use of increasingly aggressive techniques to obtain effective radicality or at least notable cytoreduction to enable possible chemotherapy to have greater efficacy. Nevertheless, some demolitions are handled with care, given that reconstruction is not always straightforward and free from complications.

Gray et al. suggested in 1996 [6] that obtaining correct and sufficient resection of soft tissue tumors of the anterior abdominal wall required the removal of the tumor *en bloc* from the wall, and that this was enabled by the possibility of reconstructing the wall with the use of polypropylene mesh.

Polypropylene mesh was also used by Puppo et al. [7] in 2005 to reconstruct pelvic floor integrity following radical cystectomy for a stage T2 bladder tumor with associated vaginal prolapse after subtotal hysterectomy, associated with an ileal reservoir for the urethra. Female incontinence and the prolapse of pelvic organs has been defined as a contraindication for orthotopic replacement of the bladder, though with this reconstruction a check-up at one year demonstrated complete day continence and the use of a pad for the night hours only.

Reconstruction following vulvar carcinoma may also be difficult, since large surgical excision is the chosen treatment for this tumor, but this can result in large losses of substance particularly in the inguinal region where radical lymphadenectomy needs to be conducted.

In 2006 Olejek [8] first proposed the use of a polypropylene mesh to protect vessels in the saphenous ostia after this procedure. The thoracic wall and the sternum are often involved in primitive or secondary tumors, the removal of which causes the problem of closing the newly-created defect.

The use of a prosthesis in pure Marlex or combined with methylmetacrylate [9] or combined with a prosthesis in stainless steel [10] have been proposed. The results seem satisfactory and the authors propose repair with this technique as the most effective for repairing defects of the thoracic area, due to secondary localizations particularly from breast carcinoma or endometrial carcinoma [11]. However, this type of mesh is not usable in all cases and presents contraindications on being placed in contact with the intestine or used in a potentially or actually infected field.

Modern technology has produced a solution for these situations, with the introduction of new biological prostheses derived from porcine or bovine collagen, with various products that differ in some of their details that might be important in particular situations.

The prostheses are composed of acellular porcine collagen and its elastin fibres. Their architecture is very similar to that of human tissue and its three-dimensional characteristic is conserved. A precise, controlled degree of cross-linking may be introduced into the structure, making it resistant to the collagenase enzymes responsible for fragmentation and reabsorption of implanted collagen. If this characteristic is introduced, the implant proves resistant over time, constituting a solid structure upon which the body reconstructs its own tissue.

These implants prove to be resistant to infections and have as their main indication use in contaminated and potentially or actually infected fields. Another indication may be obtained from the work of Murphy and Corbally [12].

The reconstruction of defects of the wall in subjects still developing may not be conducted with inert materials that maintain their structure over time, as they tend to prevent growth of the structure they are intended to repair. The example of reconstruction of the thoracic wall with the implantation of a non cross-linked biological prosthesis following removal of a Ewing tumor in the paediatric population is highly indicative and suggestive for the new possibilities it offers.

The reconstruction of organs liable to variations in volume may also become an important indication: for example, the reconstruction of the vagina following pelvic exenteration for gynecological tumors [13].

The intrinsic features of these prostheses suggest a use not yet reported in the literature, but which may become interesting: following abdominoperineal rectal amputation according to Miles, an empty pelvic space is created where intestinal loops may be inserted, making subsequent radiotherapy risky for the integrity of the loops themselves, as well as the increase in the risk of occlusion due to volvulus or torsion. This has been avoided to date with omentum-plasty when possible, or with the use of resorbable prostheses in Vicryl or non-resorbable in PTFE. However, these solutions have not proved to be optimal, either as they are impracticable (little omentum or need for omentectomy) or because they are prone to subsequent complications like superinfections or adherences that cause intestinal occlusion.

The use of a biological prosthesis to create a pelvic neo-diaphragm with the aim of isolating the zone to be radiated from the overlying intestinal loops and rendering it immune to infections and adherences might reveal itself to be the ideal solution for enabling the application of multimodal treatment for the rectal tumor, which certainly offers greater advantages than surgery alone.

Of course these new possibilities allow oncological surgeons to tackle tumor disease with a more aggressive attitude and obtain a result ever closer to radicality, knowing they have at their disposal aids fit to ensure satisfactory reconstruction and

4

thus permitting the subsequent radio- or chemotherapy treatment to have greater efficacy and consequently a more favorable impact in terms of survival and recurrence.

Surgery for Wall Defects

The incidence of incisional hernias following laparotomy varies from 2–11% up to 16% in some case series [14]. Predisposing factors do not, however, seem to include tumor disease, even if in the studies reported in the literature postoperative adjuvant chemotherapy is not considered a risk factor. Chronic obstructive pulmonary disease, wound infections and diabetes are, on the other hand, significantly correlated with the onset of postoperative incisional hernias [14,15]. Higher incidence occurs in the first year after the operation, though with the increase in survival due to the progress in operating techniques and adjuvant chemotherapy hernias that arise at three, five or ten years after surgical treatment are not rare. Nutritional factors (cachexia, malnutrition or malabsorption) have not be correlated with this disease.

The oncological surgeon is therefore faced with two types of problem to tackle: the surgical treatment of tumors with hernias of the wall already present and the treatment of subsequent hernias based on life expectancy and the modalities of reconstruction available.

In the case of an already present hernia and the need to treat a tumor with a potentially contaminated operation (colon tumors, abscessualized, perforated), up to some time ago a prosthesis could not be used given the risk of infection and failure of the wall reconstruction. Recourse to alternative techniques for freeing components of the abdominal wall (Ramirez) might give guarantees of success that were not optimal, though they enabled the oncological operation, reserving for a possible further operation the treatment of a not uncommon hernia recurrence. Possible postoperative chemotherapy certainly did not favor, moreover, scar-tissue healing.

The positioning of a retromuscular mesh might be attempted in the case of low contamination of the surgical field, though bearing clearly in mind the risks run of infection in these cases.

The realization of new biological prostheses offers an optimal solution for these cases. Their resistance to infections and their static support function for genetic collagen reconstruction of the body enable their use also in cases of free peritonitis or the presence of clearly infected material [16]. They also permit radical operations including demolition of part of the abdominal wall, supplying the surgeon with reliable material to use in reconstruction, and permitting treatment of the defect in the wall at the same time as oncological treatment. Their use is currently spreading and the European Hernia Society has created the European Registry for Biological Prostheses which is a prospective registry on the use of collagen biological prostheses in (potentially) infected fields. This registry will collect the data from 2008 to December 2010 concerning the preoperative conditions, indications, surgical procedure and results at one month and one year.

Knowing that these new aids are available, the dilemma arises whether or not to operate on an incisional hernia in a tumor patient. The extension of survival that has been obtained with modern surgery techniques and radio-chemotherapy support brings to our notice many incisional hernias in tumor patients. Their treatment, which does not differ normally from that of other post-laparotomy hernias, may nevertheless be a source of doubt at the moment of analyzing the patient's life expectancy.

The ethical dilemma is whether it is fair and correct to treat a post-laparotomy hernia when life expectancy is lower than 6 months – 1 year, and whether the corrective operation entails a delay in beginning chemotherapy treatment. Our attitude is that if quality of life without repair is decidedly poor, then the operation should be taken into consideration, but the technique to be used should be the least invasive possible, though maintaining good efficacy. Thus it will not be decided to use highly expensive mesh if life expectancy is lower than one year but alternative techniques may be chosen that could eventually give a higher relapse percentage in the first year, though perhaps this recurrence will not unfortunately have the time to become manifest. However, even with poor expectancy the quality of life must be improved, so if the clinical and physical conditions of the patient enable it and their motivation is strong, the patient must be operated on.

The new concept of mesh in low cost material (polypropylene) and low weight provides excellent materials for treating post-laparotomy hernias with traditional techniques (Rives) and with satisfactory results in terms of success and patient compliance[17]. The use of human fibrin-based glues for fixing them also reduces the discomfort created when stitches are used, adding a relatively small cost to the operation in the face of decidedly favorable results [18].

Surgery for Inguinal Hernia

The treatment of an inguinal, crural or umbilical hernia, which currently can be carried out with minimally invasive surgery under local anesthetic in most cases and almost always with patient discharge on the same day as the operation (day-surgery), allows the surgeon to easily remedy this disorder which is often the cause of functional limitations and painful and particularly invalidating symptoms in the oncological patient. High grading of the treatment, the limited costs, and above all the ability to improve the residual quality of life beyond prognostic forecasts of tumor disease impose careful evaluation of this therapeutic opportunity on the part of carers, which, moreover, if correctly applied proves to be conclusive.

While also bearing in mind the possible risk of complications such as the strangled or obstructed hernia which this disease can cause and which in patients of this type can be particularly serious, the arguments above must be considered all the more seriously also on the part of the person suffering from the problems which a negative event of this nature might determine. Although the traumas involved in hernioplasty are limited, the benefits which can be brought by its implementation should however be related to the histological type and stage of the tumor, its site, age, general clinical conditions, and any presence of aggravating factors such as ascites, patient build and personality. Thus establishing *a priori* indication and timing of its execution with respect to oncological (surgical or not) care that the tumor requires and to which precedence should be given is not always possible.

The in-depth analysis of all the elements connected with the entity of the principal disease and disorders suffered due to the hernia should not lead to simplistic or hurried considerations concerning vital decisions, confirming the need of a multidisciplinary approach for the cancer. Moreover, the possibility of combining the oncological operations (carried out both with a radical intent and for a palliative purpose) with the concomitant hernia repair has become realistic in many situations. Although not often proposed and perhaps also debatable up until relatively recent times, this simultaneous execution, which has the current support of clinical results, may be taken into consideration also in the case of highly complex surgical procedures and those with a high probability of contamination like those concerning intestinal tumors.

The implementation of an operation that is "not clean" would make a simultaneous hernioplasty inadvisable, forbidding 'tailoring' with the usual prosthetic meshes for reasons that can been imagined connected with a possible infection. Nevertheless, even if plausible, all this is only partially true due to the evolution that the materials used have undergone in recent years. New composition prostheses, other fully biological prostheses made up of bovine collagen, light meshes or meshes which are resorbable by the body after implantation, or combined with non-stick substances, and lastly the use of aids like adhesives able to secure the prostheses without suture are all innovations able to disprove past statements questioning the ability of the prosthesis to be held safely in place and the risk of complications in the field of sepsis, and able to achieve a high percentage of success.

For these intrinsic characteristics, in cases where deep repair proves necessary, the operative technique may also envisage "underlay" placing, namely in a retromuscular position, in the pre-peritoneal sphere or the abdominal cavity itself in close contact with the loops, together with the removal of the intestinal tract affected by the tumor.

Above all in the elderly patient, an inguinal hernia may sometimes reveal the presence of an unacknowledged carcinoma of the colon, acting as a sign of tumor disease. Thanks to the new finds, also in this setting the simultaneous double operation of colon resection and plastic surgery of the wall is feasible in the same way as may take place in the presence of a voluminous hernial swelling combined with a benign disease of an inflammatory type like diverticulitis.

In the light of these facts, new routes able to modify the therapeutic conduct for a hernia of the abdomen associated with a tumor appear as pathways mainly due to the new instruments at the surgeon's disposal. The need for a "reinforcement patch" in hernia repair and the recent development of new prostheses is confirmation of the direction in which modern research will have to address its efforts in the coming years. In particular the total absence of intrusion of synthetic materials foreign to the body for hernioplasty, and with the aid of supporting nanotechnology for the framework upon which the new reinforcement tissue will be able to be built, may in the future represent the gold standard of care for this common disorder especially if combined with an illness still in many ways obscure and with many unknown features.

References

1. Vasiliev JuM, Moizhess TG (1982) Tumorigenicity of sarcoma cells is enhanced by the local environment of implanted foreign body. Int J Cancer. 30:525–529
2. Brand KG, Buoen LC, Johnson KH, Brand I (1975) Etiological factors, stages, and the role of the foreign body in foreign body tumorigenesis: a review. Cancer Res 35:279–286
3. Jennings TA, Peterson L, Axiotis CA et al (1988) Angiosarcoma associated with foreign body material. A report of three cases. Cancer 62:2436–2444
4. Ghadimi BM, Langer C, Becker H (2002) The carcinogenic potential of biomaterials in hernia surgery. Chirurg 73:833–837
5. Imai M, Kondo Y, Masuko H et al (2003) Distant peritoneal metastasis to a mesh-plug prosthesis in a gastrointestinal cancer patient: report of a case. Surg Today 33:864–866
6. Gray MW, Caleel RT, Sorg RJ (1996) Soft tissue sarcoma of the anterior abdominal wall: review of reconstruction techniques. J Am Osteopath Assoc 96:48–53
7. Puppo P, Introini C, Calvi P, Naselli A (2005) Pelvic floor reconstruction before orthotopic bladder replacement after radical cystectomy for bladder cancer. Urology 65:174
8. Olejek A (2006) Use of prolene mesh in surgical treatment of tissue defects after radical inguinal and pelvic lymph node dissection in vulvar cancer–a brief report. Int J Gynecol Cancer 16:448–451
9. Akan M, Eker Uluçay G, Kargi B et al (2006) Combined reconstruction of complex defects of the chest wall. Scand J Plast Reconstr Surg Hand Surg 40:93–100
10. Haraguchi S, Hioki M, Hisayoshi T et al (2006) Resection of sternal tumors and reconstruction of the thorax: a review of 15 patients. Surg Today 36:225–229
11. Haraguchi S, Hioki M, Hisayoshi T et al (2006) Resection of sternal metastasis from endometrial carcinoma followed by reconstruction with sandwiched marlex and stainless steel mesh: report of a case. Surg Today 36:184–186
12. Murphy F, Corbally MT (2007) The novel use of small intestinal submucosal matrix for chest wall reconstruction following Ewing's tumor resection. Pediatr Surg Int 23:353–356
13. Rettenmaier MA, Goldstein BH, Micha JP, Brown JV (2006) Vaginal reconstruction following supra-levator total pelvic exenteration. Gynecol Oncol 102:397–399
14. Adell-Carceller R, Segarra-Soria MA, Pellicer-Castell V et al (2006) Incisional hernia in colorectal cancer surgery. Associated risk factors. Cir Esp 79:42–45
15. Franchi M, Ghezzi F, Buttarelli M et al (2001) Incisional hernia in gynecologic oncology patients: a 10-year study. Obstet Gynecol 97:696–700
16. Shaikh FM, Giri SK, Durrani S et al (2007) Experience with porcine acellular dermal collagen implant in one-stage tension-free reconstruction of acute and chronic abdominal wall defects. World J Surg 31:1966–1972
17. Trombetta F, Tonda-Turo C, Tori A (2008) Light- and heavy-weight meshes: comparison of two concepts. Osp Ital Chir 14:88–94
18. Kingsnorth AN, Shahid MK, Valliattu AJ et al (2008) Open onlay mesh repair for major abdominal wall hernias with selective use of components separation and fibrin sealant. World J Surg 32:26–30

Intraoperative Radiotherapy

5

U. Ricardi, M. Rampino, A. Reali, B. Mussa, P. Marsanic

Intraoperative radiotherapy (IORT) is the delivery of a single large radiation dose to the tumor bed during surgical resection. This radiation modality is applied in association with surgery and external beam radiotherapy (EBRT) or chemotherapy in the treatment of locally advanced cancer of the abdomen, pelvis, neck, cranium, thorax and extremities [1] with the final goal of enhancing locoregional tumor control [2].The initial clinical use of IORT dates back to the early 1900s, when IORT was performed using soft X-rays and moving patients from the operating room to the radiotherapy bunker. The first IORT using electron beams (IOERT) was carried out in November 1976 at Howard University, in a bunker equipped with an operating room. In the 1980s, in order to combine technical advantages of brachytherapy with logistic advantages of IORT, high dose rate brachytherapy IORT (HDR-IORT) was implemented at Memorial Sloan-Kettering Cancer Center, using a portable HDR machine (OMIT) [2, 3].Since the 1990s dedicated linear accelerators have been created to solve IORT logistical problems. Currently, 220 mobile units are installed worldwide: 40% in the United States, 35% in Europe and 25% in Japan. There are three principal models used in clinical practice [4]: Mobetron, from "Intraop Medical Incorporated", California USA, Novac7 (Fig. 5.1), from "New Radiant Technology", Italy and Liac from "Sordina", Italy. These machines are small linear accelerators producing electron beams which can be positioned directly in the existing operating rooms, with no special shielding required [5]. Lastly, the Intrabeam Photon Radiosurgery System (Zeiss Inc, Germany) is used for breast cancer treatment [6]: it is a miniature electron beam-driven X-ray source that provides a point source of low-energy X-ray (50 kV maximum) at the tip of a 3.2 mm diameter tube. Several professionals from different disciplines are involved in IORT management for patient selection and clinical application and so the report of Task Force 48 of the Radiation Therapy Committee American Association of Physicists in Medicine

U. Ricardi (✉)
Oncologic Radiotherapy Unit, S. Giovanni Battista University Hospital, Turin, Italy

New Technologies in Surgical Oncology. Antonio Mussa (Ed.)
© Springer-Verlag Italia 2010

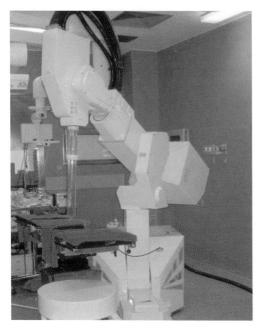

Fig. 5.1 Novac 7 mobile linear accelerator

suggests instituting an IORT team in every IORT centre [1]. The members of the IORT team should be:

1. The surgeon
2. The radiation oncologist
3. The radiation physicist
4. The radiotherapy technologist
5. The anesthesiologist
6. The nursing staff

The *surgeon* discusses clinical cases and the best surgical procedure with radiation oncologist and co-operates in setting up the patient during IORT [1, 7].

The *radiation oncologist* is clinically responsible for prescription and delivery of treatment [7] and decides on IORT dose, field size, beam energy and technical approach according to disease extension and the closeness to organs at risk. Along with the surgeon and the radiotherapy technologist, the radiation oncologist is responsible for the "docking" procedure.

The *radiation physicist* is responsible for dosimeter data acquisition and for machine quality control. It is important that radiation physicists have dosimeters data readily available to calculate the monitor units required to deliver an adequate dose-prescription.

The *radiotherapy technologist* is the professional profile dedicated to the mobilization of the IORT accelerator during docking procedure and to deliver the dose prescribed by the radiation oncologist. Radiotherapy technologist is responsible for irradiation data registration and co-operates for quality assurance treatment.

The *anesthesiologist* must control the patient's vital signs during irradiation through a remote system or by closed-circuit television; rapid access into treatment room is required to attend to patient in any instance.

The *nursing staff* of the operating room have responsibilities before, during and after the IORT procedure. Preoperatively the role includes applicator sterility assurance, surgery planning and patient transfer. During IORT procedure nursing staff is responsible for providing support to IORT team and lastly for keeping inventory of all used applicators and returning them for sterilization.

In 1998, a new professional society, the International Society of IORT (ISIORT) was created for the scientific and clinical development of IORT. The ISIORT has now over 1000 members from more than 20 countries and a scientific meeting is organized every two years. The first ISIORT meeting was held in September 1998 in Pamplona, at the University of Navarre, one of the most famous IORT centers. In Italy, according to data collected from AIRO (Italian Association of Radiation Oncology) at the end of 2007, there are 27 centres able to administer IORT in clinical practice, with an average of 34 patients treated per year from each centre. IORT is becoming an important component of the multidisciplinary treatment approach: in literature review, pancreatic cancer, retroperitoneal soft tissues sarcomas, locally advanced and recurrent rectal cancer are evidence-based IORT indications. Now we will illustrate IORT results in these pathological settings and in an area – breast cancer – where clinical research is particularly interesting.

IORT and Pancreatic Cancer

Prognosis for pancreatic cancer remains poor with a high incidence of local relapse, even when disease is potentially resectable. In order to overcome this problem, several studies have been conducted with the delivery of IORT to the tumor bed following pancreaticoduodenectomy, showing an increase in local control [8] without a prolongation of survival [2,9,10]. Referred IORT doses are usually 10-15 Gy [10] with a range from 10 to 30 Gy [2]. The treatment field includes retroperitoneum and tumor bed while the pancreatic remnant is usually excluded. The major retroperitoneal blood vessel, i.e. aorta, celiac axis, superior mesenteric artery, superior mesenteric vein, portal vein and inferior vena cava can be included in IORT field because they are not particularly radiosensitive (Fig. 5.2). The most frequent postoperative complications are anastomotic leakage, peripancreatic abscess formation and pancreatic fistula [10]. However, IORT could offer a certain benefit in localized pancreatic cancer in combination with preoperative chemoradiation and adjuvant "modern" chemotherapy, but this approach should be tested in prospective trials [8]. In locally advanced or metastatic pancreatic cancer, there is currently no clear evidence of clinical effectiveness [10] but IORT is appreciated for the lasting effect in pain control in patients with unresectable disease [11].

5

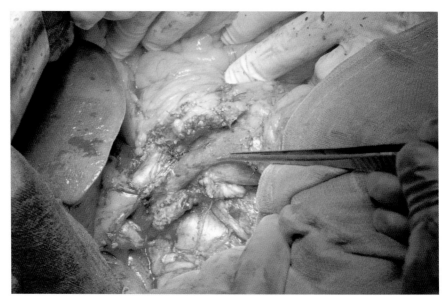

Fig. 5.2 Pancreatic cancer: tumour site after resection

IORT and Advanced and Recurrent Rectal Cancer

Isolated recurrences limited to the pelvis are the most frequent problem after resection of locally advanced rectal carcinomas, even if several studies have demonstrated that preoperative external radiation therapy (EBRT) can reduce relapse rate. IORT can be considered an ideal "boost" technique in order to obtain dose-escalation [2,6,12]; EBRT in combination with IORT, in fact, allows local delivery of a tumoricidal biological dose of up to 80-90 Gy [13]. In the same way a IORT boost can be considered for patients affected by previously irradiated recurrent rectal cancer [2,6,12,14]. In both situations, the target volume is the "higher risk area" (i.e. where the tumor is fixed or where there is a macroscopic or possible microscopic residual). In locally advanced rectal cancer as well as in recurrent rectal cancer, most studies referred an IORT median dose of 15 Gy (range 12.5–20 Gy) [2,6,12] specified on 90% isodose [2,12,13]. The most frequent complications are urinary infections and symptomatic or objective neuropathy [2]; the ureter is not a dose-limiting structure but, as ureteral narrowing or obstruction can occur, stent positioning before surgery is suggested. Peripheral nerves are the main dose-limiting structures for IORT but significantly fewer complications occur for doses of 12.5 Gy or less [15]. From the review of literature data, multimodal therapy can be proposed for patients with locally unresectable primary colorectal cancers which includes preoperative EBRT and extended surgical resection with IORT, followed by adjuvant chemotherapy. This regimen could offer excellent local disease control with low perioperative morbidity [15]; obviously randomized trials are needed. Encouraging but preliminary data exist also for IORT treatment of rectal cancer recurrences.

IORT and Retroperitoneal Soft Tissue Sarcomas

Surgery is the main treatment and provides the most favorable prognosis after complete resection (R0) but complete surgical resection is often difficult or impossible due to the anatomical location of these tumors and the frequent invasion of contiguous retroperitoneal structures [16]. In this scenario, IORT appears to be an appropriate treatment, associated with EBRT, with the aim of improving local control. Several treatment schedules have been studied including preoperative or postoperative EBRT associated with IORT. Although there is no doubt about the benefit from adjuvant EBRT, a high dose delivery in the postoperative setting is limited by the tolerance of normal structures (i.e. small intestine, kidneys, spinal cord) included in tumor bed [17]. Preoperative EBRT has theoretical advantages, e.g. treating tumor "in situ" clearly facilitates RT-planning and there is also the possibility of converting unresectable diseases to complete resection [17]. Several retrospective studies suggest improvements in local control through the addition of adjuvant radiation [18] and some authors underline IORT role in obtaining a significant reduction in local failure [6,16,19]. IORT can be delivered prior to as well as after EBRT and the median dose is 15 Gy with a range of 10-20 Gy [2,16–18]; the target is the tumor bed with a 1-3 cm safety margin and the dose is generally prescribed on the 90% isodose. Potential side effects of intra-operative treatment are related to the site of the target volume. Neurotoxicity is the most common side effect [2,16], particularly when the IORT dose is higher than 15 Gy. Retroperitoneal abscess incidence is low while ureteral stricture may occur when ureter is included in irradiation field [2,16].

IORT and Breast Cancer

Partial breast irradiation (PBI) has been tested in limited pilot studies and seems able to provide acceptable cosmesis, minimal toxicity and adequate local control. The idea of a single-shot treatment by IOERT, as proposed by the Milan Group, is tempting especially in low risk patients, but follow-up periods far beyond 5 years are mandatory to provide definitive evidence on long-term local control rates [6,20,21]. An interesting multicentre trial of Targeted Intraoperative Radiation Therapy (TARGIT) had as principal objective to determine whether IORT targeted to tumor bed could provide equivalent local control compared with whole-breast irradiation in patients with early-stage invasive breast cancer [6,22]. A total of 779 patients were accrued from 16 institutions all over the world: obviously definitive local control data need a longer follow-up [22].

Moreover, IORT is an interesting option for patients with localized breast recurrences after previous EBRT [23]. The idea of IOERT as a "boost" strategy during breast conserving therapy in limited stage breast cancer is attractive but published data are low and rarely updated. So a recent pooled analysis was performed by 6 ISIORT-Europe institutions: 1131 patients, treated from 1998 to 2005, were studied

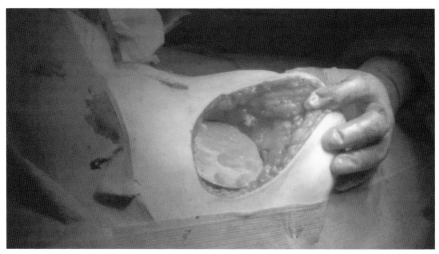

Fig. 5.3 Breast cancer: chest wall protection

and IORT as "anticipated boost" showed an optimal accuracy in dose delivery and good local tumor control rates [24]. At any rate IORT technique in breast cancer has the same procedure: after lumpectomy with satisfactory tumor-free margins dedicated aluminium-lead disks are placed above the pectoralis muscle (Fig. 5.3) in order to minimize irradiation to thoracic wall. Then mammary parenchyma is sutured in surgery breach area and target volume thickness is measured. Finally an applicator of proper diameter is placed in tumor bed (Fig. 5.4) and sterile gauze are positioned between skin and applicator's edge. Optimal energy is selected on the basis of measured target thickness. Dose varies according to treatment "rationale" (single shot versus boost) and is prescribed on 90% isodose [6].

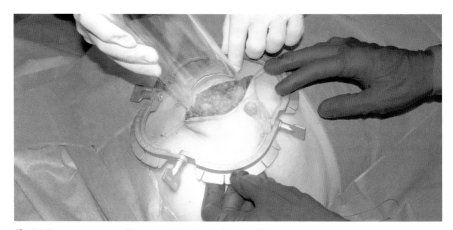

Fig. 5.4 Breast cancer: applicator positioning before docking

References

1. Palta JR, Biggs PJ, Hazle JD et al (1995) Intraoperative electron beam radiation therapy: technique, dosimetry, and dose specification: report of task force 48 of the radiation therapy committee, american association of physicists in medicine. Int J Rad Oncol Biol Phys 33:725–746
2. Gunderson LL, Willet CG, Harrison LB, Calvo FA (1999) Intraoperative irradiation. Techniques and results. Humana Press, Totowa, New Jersey
3. Calvo FA, Meirino RM, Orecchia R (2006) Intraoperative radiation therapy. First part: rationale and techniques. Crit Rev Oncol Hematol 59:106–115
4. Beddar AS, Biggs PJ, Chang S et al (2006) Intraoperative radiation therapy using mobile electron linear accelerators: Report of AAPM Radiation Therapy Committee Task Group No. 72. Med Phys 33:1476–1489
5. Daves JL, Mills MD (2001) Shielding assessment of a mobile electron accelerator for intraoperative radiotherapy. J Appl Clin Med Phys 2:165–173
6. Calvo FA, Meirino RM, Orecchia R (2006) Intraoperative radiation therapy. Part 2: Clinical results. Crit Rev Oncol Hematol 59:116–127
7. Istituto Superiore della Sanità (2003) Linee guida per la garanzia di qualità nella radioterapia intraoperatoria. Rapporti ISTISAN 03/1 IT
8. Valentini V, Moranti AG, Macchia G et al (2008) Intraoperative radiation therapy in resected pancreatic carcinoma: long-term analysis. Int J Rad Oncol Biol Phys 70:1094–1099
9. Hiraoka T, Kanemitsu K (1999) Value of extended resection and intraoperative radiotherapy for resectable pancreatic cancer. World J Surg 23:930–936
10. Ruano-Ravina A, Almazán Ortega R, Guedea F (2008) Intraoperative radiotherapy in pancreatic cancer: a systematic review. Radiother Oncol 87:318–325
11. Calvo FA, Valentini V (2008) Radiotherapy for pancreatic cancer: Systematic nihilism or intraoperative realism. Radiother Oncol 87:314–317
12. Wiig JN, Poulsen JP, Tveit KM et al (2000) Intra-operative irradiation (IORT) for primary advanced and recurrent rectal cancer: a need for randomised studies. Eur J Cancer 36:868–874
13. Dresen RC, Gosen MJ, Martijn H et al (2008) Radical resection after IORT-containing multimodality treatment is the most important determinant for outcome in patients treated for locally recurrent rectal cancer. Ann Surg Oncol 15:1937–1947
14. Pezner RD, Chu DZJ, Ellenhorn JDI (2002) Intraoperative radiation therapy for patients with recurrent rectal cancer and sigmoid colon cancer in previously irradiated fields. Radiother Oncol 64:47–52
15. Mathis KL, Nelson H, Pemberton JH et al (2008) Unresectable colorectal cancer can be cured with multimodality therapy. Ann Surg 284:592–598
16. Bobin JY, Al-Lawati T, Granero LE et al (2003) Surgical management of retroperitoneal sarcomas associated with external and intraoperative electron beam radiotherapy. Eur J Surg Oncol 29:676–681
17. Caudle AS, Tepper JE, Calvo BF et al (2006) Complications associated with neoadjuvant radiotherapy in the multidisciplinary treatment of retroperitoneal sarcomas. Ann Surg Oncol 14:577–582
18. Ballo MT, Zagars GK, Pollock RE et al (2007) Retroperitoneal soft tissue sarcoma: an analysis of radiation and surgical treatment. Int J Rad Oncol Biol Phys 67:158–163
19. Sindelar WF, Kinsella TJ, Chen PW et al (1993) Intraoperative radiotherapy in retroperitoneal sarcomas: final results of a prospective, randomized, clinical trial. Arch Surg 128:402–410
20. Veronesi U, Orecchia R, Luini A et al (2005) Full-dose intraoperative radiotherapy with electrons during breast-conserving surgery: experience with 590 cases. Ann Surg 242:101–106
21. Sacchini V, Beal K, Goldberg J et al (2008) Study of quadrant high-dose intraoperative radiation therapy for early-stage breast cancer. Br J Surg 95:1105–1110

5

22. Holmes DR, Baum M, Joseph D (2007) The TARGIT trial: targeted intraoperative radiation therapy versus conventional postoperative whole-breast radiotherapy after breast-conserving surgery for the management of early-stage invasive breast cancer (a trial update). Am J Surg 194:507–510

23. Kraus-Tiefenbacher U, Bauer L, Scheda A et al (2007) Intraoperative radiotherapy (IORT) is an option for patients with localized breast recurrences after previous external-beam radiotherapy. BMC Cancer 14:178

24. Sedlmayer F, Faster G, Merz F et al on behalf of the ISIORT Europe (2007) IORT with electrons as a boost strategy during breast conserving therapy in limited stage breast cancer: results of an ISIORT pooled analysis. Strahlenther Onkol 183:32–34

New Technologies in Oncological Endocrine Surgery

6

M. Deandrea, A. Mobiglia, E. Brignardello

Endocrine surgery is an extremely heterogeneous sphere as regards organ involvement and different therapeutic approaches, even in the oncological field alone. In this chapter all innovations which may be considered technical and technological in nature and which have passed through recent surgical practice in oncology will be systematically examined, while attempting to methodically maintain order for each organ.

Technical Innovations in the Field of Thyroid Surgery

The approach to known tumor disease of the thyroid has been standardized for some time at the best known surgery centres at international level, and the surgical procedures optimized to the point that they differ very little – except perhaps in procedure times and indexes of complications – for the expert operators in the sector.

In the last ten years, however, the adoption in selected cases of a mini-invasive surgical approach to neoplastic thyroid disease has made it possible to perform the procedure with greater respect for the esthetic elements of a zone, i.e. the front of the neck, which is so important for relational life.

Considering that the current limits of preoperative diagnosis of differentiated carcinoma of the thyroid are connected with the difficulty of detecting follicular forms via FNAB cytology, even when performed with the help of immunohistochemical tests, such as anti-Galectin 3 antibody staining (around 20% of nodes subjected to needle aspiration present a cytological diagnosis of "follicular neoformation", but only 20% of these prove to be malignant when the surgical specimen is histologically tested), subjecting patients to surgical verification in such circumstances cannot be avoided.

M. Deandrea (✉)
Oncological Endocrine Surgery Service, S. Giovanni Battista University Hospital, Turin, Italy

New Technologies in Surgical Oncology. Antonio Mussa (Ed.)
© Springer-Verlag Italia 2010

53

6

In the third millennium we are trying to establish diagnostic potential with methods alternative to the surgical procedure and with less impact for the patient. However, if this is not possible, diagnostic surgery is sometimes still indicated, with the aim of obtaining when possible an option with efficacious therapeutic value. With the intention of making this aspect tolerable, the indication of mini-invasive (MIVAT) techniques has been extended in the oncological field (Table 6.1).

This procedure has had an appreciably different approach throughout the world produced by dissimilar habits and the multiple skills of individual operators (Table 6.2) [1–6]. Nevertheless, over the course of the years there has been a convergence in the area of video-assisted techniques without pneumo-neck, with a direct approach in the anterior region [7].

Table 6.1 Current indications and contraindications for MIVAT

Indications
- Thyroid nodules with diameter less than 3-3.5 cm
- Indeterminate cytology
- Follicular lesions
- "Low risk" papillary carcinoma
- Basedow's disease with gland not exceeding 20 ml
- Prophylactic thyroidectomy in patients who are carriers of RET gene mutation

Contraindications
- History of thyroiditis (positive antibodies)
- Previous neck irradiation
- Previous thyroid or parathyroid surgery

Table 6.2 Proposed techniques for mini-invasive surgery for thyroid disease

Type of access	Reference
Videoscopic lateral supraclavicular according to Gagner	Br J Surg 83:875; 1996 [1]
Videoscopic lateral cervical according to Henry	Langenbecks Arch Surg 384:298; 1999 [2]
Video-assisted cervical according to Shimizu	J Am Coll Surg 188:697; 1999 [3]
Videoscopic axillary according to Ikeda	J Am Coll Surg 191:336; 2000 [4]
Mammary according to Ohgami	Surg Laparosc Endosc Perc Tech 10:1; 2000 [5]
Video-assisted central cervical (MIVAT) according to Miccoli	J Endocrinol Investigation 20:429; 1997 [6]

In particular, this surgical approach has been made possible and has become quite widespread thanks to manageable systems of coagulation and section, which have reduced the use of metal clips or laces. This has made dissection and obliteration of vascular pedicles just as safe, rapid and efficacious, almost determining potentially "sutureless" thyroidectomy, and has been coupled with optical devices of ever smaller dimensions so as to allow reassuring control of the operative field through an incision of around 2 cm. The results of application of these techniques are given in Table 6.3.

The hemostasis technology (Table 6.4) used in this field has been extended to applications in traditional surgery, too, partly supplanting the use of bipolar cauterization (introduced by Greenwood in 1940). Currently both methods most recently proposed, the ultrasound and the radiofrequency dissector, compete in the operating theatre to produce maximum hemostatic safety, optimization of operating times and stability of results.

Table 6.3 Results of MIVAT technique operators according to Miccoli

Lobectomy mean operation time	20–120 min
Thyroidectomy mean operation time	30–130 min
Conversion to traditional	2–5% of cases
Temporary paralysis inferior laryngeal nerve	2.6%
Definitive paralysis inferior laryngeal nerve	1.1%
Transitory hypoparathyroidism	2.9%
Definitive hypoparathyroidism	0.2%
Post-operative hemorrhage	0.2%

Table 6.4 Ultrasound and radiofrequency dissection and coagulation: comparison of features

Principle	Modality	Effect	Action temperatures	Lateral thermal diffusion	Advantages of aids currently on market for use in thyroid field
Ultrasound	Mechanical vibration	Protein denaturation and coagulation	50–100°C	2 mm	CS14, Harmonic Focus Coagulation and contemporary section
Radiofrequency	Bipolar type electric field	Fusion of collagen and elastin	60–70°C	1–3 mm	Ligasure Precise Manipulation manageability

6

The sentinel lymph node (SLN) concept in the field of endocrine surgery has recently been introduced; the applicative aims for differentiated thyroid tumors have been discussed by different schools of surgery, however, and, guided by the importance of its application in the case of breast carcinoma, it has also been proposed in this context. The ultimate aim is to modulate lymph node dissection of the central compartment based on the extemporary outcome of the SLN, thus offering a potential contribution to the indication of possible radiometabolic treatment, in the case of positivity, although currently this option has not been validated.

Two principal agents exist that are used for the execution of lymph node-lymphatic localization: vital dyes and radioactive tracers. The results of the most recent studies published in the literature appear promising for both methods, one certainly encumbered by the need to perform the tracer injection in a nuclear-medical protected environment, and the other potentially problematic due to confusing permeation of the vital dye above all for peri-lesional instillations (Table 6.5) [8–11].

The same technology seems to offer a potential contribution also in terms of increased diagnostic capacity of the operator in the event of sub-clinical neoplastic recurrences, through the applications of the radioguided occult lesion localization technique also in thyroid surgery [12]. This technique was developed to seek, identify and remove non-palpable masses and has been applied mostly in the field of breast surgery; nevertheless initial reports are present in the literature of application in the case of locoregional recurrence of differentiated carcinoma of the thyroid with the aim of finding suspicious nodal or scar localizations at US evaluation, but clinically not detectable. Localization envisages the use of nuclear-medical methods: in particular, the suspicious lesion is localized by high frequency ultrasound and suitable quantities of albumin macroaggregate marked with ^{99}Tc are injected directly into the tissue suspected of recurrence; the tissue, thus marked, is removed under the guidance of a manual gamma-ray probe.

Research in the oncological sphere then considers future possibilities of treating lesions, in subjects not amenable to an ablative surgical procedure due to high-risk concomitant disease, by thermoablation with radiofrequency or laser [13–16].

Table 6.5 Application of sentinel lymph node (SLN) research in the sphere of differentiated thyroid tumors

Method	N patients	Injection site	SLN location	SLN + for metastasis	Author (year)
Isosulphan blue	103	intratumoral	100%	37%	Kim (2006) [8]
Patent blue	153	intratumoral	70%	34%	Pelizzo (2006) [9]
99Tc-Nanocoll	41	intratumoral	100%	52%	Pelizzo (2006) [9]
99Tc-Nanocoll	64	peritumoral	97%	22%	Carcoforo (2007) [10]
Methylene blue	25	peritumoral	88%	86%	Wang (2007) [11]

Radiofrequency ablation is a treatment already in use to manage many neoplasms, as carcinoma of the liver, hepatic metastasis, bone metastasis and renal tumor; recently its efficacy and safety were also assessed in the treatment of nodular thyroid disease, in subjects not referable to surgery due to a high operative risk or who expressly refused surgical treatment. The data available in the literature highlight its potential application, with appreciable reductions in volume persisting 30–60 days after the procedure and improvement above all in compressive symptoms.

Laser ablation of nodular thyroid formations through the skin has been applied both in the oncological field and for the treatment of hyperfunctioning adenomas. This technique does not seem to be efficacious in the long-term control of hyperthyroidism sustained by a hyperfunctioning autonomous thyroid adenoma and therefore is not a valid alternative to radiometabolic therapy with iodine. Conversely, in the oncological field ablation with the laser technique seems efficacious in obtaining a rapid reduction in tumor mass before chemotherapy and/or radiotherapy of a thyroid carcinoma not susceptible to surgical resection or radiometabolic ablation with iodine [16].

High-energy shock waves have been used since the beginning of the 1980s in lithotripsy. The acquisition of new instruments, able to modulate the shock-wave energy in a more satisfactory manner has enabled the biological effects induced by this technology to be exploited to a maximum. With low energy, cellular proliferation and differentiation is obtained along with an increase in vascularization, whereas with high energy an acceleration of the processes leading to natural death of the cells (apoptosis) is observed. More recently, applications of this technology have been tested which appear able to open up new perspectives in the oncological field. In particular, some research projects have taken on the aim of verifying a method of anti-tumor therapy that will enable a greater cytostatic effect to be obtained with notably reduced doses of chemotherapy drugs compared with those adopted in common treatment plans. Ultimately it is hoped that a clearly superior therapeutic index can be ensured – with a drastic reduction in the dose-dependent toxic effects of the chemotherapy drug – thanks to the possibility of selectively focalizing the high energy shock waves at the tumor lesion level and significantly increasing "penetration" of the actual drug into the neoplastic cells [17].

Another innovative technique proposed for the treatment of differentiated thyroid carcinomas aims at recovering the efficacy of radiometabolic therapy with iodine in tumors which have dedifferentiated (5–20%) and have thus lost the capacity to concentrate 131-I. In the process of cell dedifferentiation some of the specific functional characteristics of the thyrocyte are actually lost. Among these the NIS (sodium/iodine "symporter"), essential for transporting iodine into the thyrocyte, takes on particular clinical importance: in the absence of NIS, in fact, radiometabolic treatment cannot be carried out, which entails a clear worsening of the prognosis. It has recently been demonstrated that valproic acid (VPA), a drug used for over 40 years for treating epilepsy, induces tumor cell differentiation both in vitro and in vivo. This effect, which is already evident at the hematic concentrations usually reached in treating generalized epilepsy, is due to the inhibitory activity of VPA on histone deacetylases. VPA induces the expression and correct localization of NIS in papillary tumor cell cultures that have experienced dedifferentiation and this translates effectively into an increased capacity of cells to pick up the radioiodine [18]. In spite of the promising experimental presuppositions, the results of the pilot clinical trials have been disappointing up to now.

The possibility appears more promising of using VPA in treatment combined with other chemotherapy drugs, with the purpose of enhancing their biological effect and reducing toxicity. The theoretic assumption exploits the effect of histone deacetylase inhibitors both on chromatin conformational changes, making the DNA more accessible to molecular action carrying out their work through damage to the DNA itself [19], and on the state of tubulin acetylation, on which the stabilization of the micro-tubules that carry out a key role in cell division processes depends [20].

Technical Innovations in the Field of Parathyroid Surgery

In recent literature it has been demonstrated that in the majority of cases of primary hyperparathyroidism (80-90%) a single parathyroid adenoma was responsible for the disease. However, the glands may quite frequently be localized in atypical sites (with bilateral exploration it is possible to single out three parathyroids in 87%, while four glands are visualized only in 45% of cases), and localization of the pathological one may consequently be difficult.

The proposal (made by Norman in 1996) was to use an isotopic tracer, sestamibi, pre-operatively and intra-operatively with the purpose of localizing the site of the adenoma and then carry out a mini-invasive radio-guided parathyroidectomy.

With the aim of performing an extremely efficient, targeted maneuver, rigid inclusion and exclusion criteria are needed (Table 6.6).

Further confirmation of the adequacy of the parathyroidectomy, at the end of the procedure, can be supplied by the intra-operative dosage of parathormone.

Like all the other radioguided surgery techniques, in this particular application strict and competent collaboration is required between surgeon, nuclear-medicine physician and pathologist to obtain the best results possible.

The procedure may also be carried out under local anesthesia, as widely published by Lo Gerfo, with different types of cervical plexus block [21] and recently proposed again by Miccoli for his personal minimally invasive parathyroidectomy technique.

Table 6.6 Inclusion and exclusion criteria for radio-guided parathyroidectomy

Inclusion criteria
- Parathyroid scintigraphy with sestamibi documenting uptake of a single gland
Exclusion criteria
- Lack of visualization of parathyroids in preoperative imaging
- Demonstration of 2 or more enlarged glands at scintigraphy and/or ECT
- Concomitant presence of thyroid nodule disease
- Positive family medical history for MEN or IPT

Technical Innovations in the Field of Adrenal Surgery

The laparoscopic adrenalectomy technique was first described by Gagner at the beginning of the 1990s. Since then this procedure has systematically become established as the alternative to conventional surgery for the treatment of surgical disease of the adrenal gland, even becoming the therapeutic standard for some indications (Table 6.7).

The technical approach envisages two substantial variables: video-adrenalectomy with an anterior transperitoneal approach and the retroperitoneal posterior one; experiences in the literature are preponderant for the anterior access.

The laparoscopic approach has significantly reduced some of the complications or consequences of conventional surgery (such as paralytic ileum, respiratory problems, infections and wound complications), without however modifying the rate of thromboembolic disease, due to the high intra-abdominal pressure connected with CO_2 insufflation, though mitigated by early mobilization of the patient.

Among the complications of laparoscopic adrenalectomy, intra- or postoperative hemorrhage is certainly the most frequent (two-thirds of global complications) and the accidental lesion of large vessels is the main cause of laparotomic conversion. The most feared complication for oncological aims is undoubtedly adrenal capsule lesion with dispersion of glandular tissue, a situation which proves decisive in the choice of surgical approach in particular in suspected adrenal carcinoma, pheochromocytoma and the case of extremely large myelolipoma.

Table 6.7 Indications and contraindications for adrenal laparoscopic surgery

Indications
- Functioning benign tumors of small dimensions
- Aldosteronomas
- Cushing's Syndrome induced by cortisol producing adrenal adenoma or bilateral hyperplasia
- Non-functioning incidentalomas of small dimensions (however >3.5–4 cm)
- Primitive tumors including suspected malignancy without signs of infiltration
Relative contraindications (connected with the tumor)
- Tumors of large dimensions (>12–14 cm)
- Pheochromocytoma (due to risk of bleeding or anesthesiological problems)
- Malignant tumors (risk of capsular breakage or "spillage")
- Rapidly growing myelolipomas, large dimensions, compressing neighboring organs
Relative contraindications (connected with the patient)
- Obesity
- Previous surgery for nephrectomy or duodenopancreatectomy
Absolute contraindications
- Contraindications for pneumoperitoneum, coagulopathy, serious cardiopulmonary disease
- Malignant tumors with signs of infiltration

Robotic surgery is the new technological challenge [22] and has been coupled nowadays, thanks to technological progress, with image fusion techniques with intra-operative video-laparoscopic visualization aimed at improving surgical orientation. This sector of clinical research requires, however, a different approach compared with conventional surgical procedures, given that the surgeon no longer has direct perception of the patient's internal organs and instead manipulates them through devices which give little or no manual feedback. Modern technology offers with virtual reality great potential for overcoming these disadvantages, e.g., with the use of haptic interfaces in robotics (namely devices that allow a real or virtual robot to be maneuverd and tactile sensations to be received from it in response–feedback). For a similar system problems do actually arise regarding the reliability, efficacy and intuitiveness on the part of the surgeon. In order to solve all these problems a highly interdisciplinary work group is required which can unite the most recent progress in the fields of virtual reality, haptics and human-computer interface design. For this purpose reports are available in some congress abstracts relating to international consortia with competence in the fields of virtual reality and enhanced reality (a particular extension of virtual reality consisting of superimposing perceived reality on a virtual reality generated by the computer using data gathered from pre-operatively performed CT-MR-scintigraphy scans, robotics, haptics, image processing, information fusion and the human factor).

Technical Innovations in the Field of Surgery on Neuroendocrine Tumors of the Gastro-entero-pancreatic Zone

The only innovative events in the field of surgery for neuroendocrine disease of the gastro-entero-pancreatic zone, leaving aside the laparoscopic approach which has also been proposed for these neoplastic forms, are those relating to radiolocalization of the forms expressing receptors for somatostatin with the help of nuclear medical imaging.

Endocrine pancreatic tumors belong to the large group of neuroendocrine tumors (NET) of the gastro-entero-pancreatic tract, the cells of which contain enzymatic structures capable of amine precursor storage and decarboxylation, an essential process for the production of monoamine neurotransmitters like serotonin, histamine and dopamine. Moreover, these cells often express somatostatin receptors on their surface. Nuclear medical molecular imaging exploits both these characteristics to develop new tracers able to visualize these tumors. Octreotide is one of the somatostatin synthesis analogs, of which it maintains the cyclic structure but enhanced to resist degradation enzymes (half-life of 2 hours compared with <2 minutes of native somatostatin). With the aim of enabling its use in imaging, the molecule is bound to a radioactive isotope (^{111}In). The principal indications for use of Octreoscan® are summarized in Table 6.8. To these the possibility has been added of using it in the intra-operative sphere through the practice of radioguided surgery. In the literature there are many reports of clinical cases subjected to the method, some in the case of

Table 6.8 Indications for use of scintigraphy with Octreoscan®

Localization of disease in presence of biochemical data and history suspect for NET
Staging in presence of NET already known
Evaluation of presence of receptors for somatostatin envisaging targeted therapy (also radiometabolic)
Monitoring of therapeutic efficacy (after surgery, radiotherapy, chemotherapy)
Follow up of patients already treated for NET

NET, Neuroendocrine tumor

functioning NET (insulinomas) [23,24], and others in the case of recurrences [25]. One element that these reports have in common is the favorable localization of the lesion even if of small dimensions, the relative certainty of radicality subsequent to radioguided removal or in the context of scar tissue, as in the case of recurrence.

Radiolabelled somatostatin analogs can also be used with therapeutic aims. Radiometabolic therapy has shown itself to be particularly useful in controlling the symptoms associated with functioning neuroendocrine tumors and is indicated in cases of widespread disease, not surgically treatable or in chemo-resistance conditions. For this aim labelled compounds with beta-emitting isotopes such as $^{90}Y(\text{-DOTA-TOC})$ or ^{177}Lu are used.

References

1. Gagner M (1996) Endoscopic parathyroidectomy (Letter). Br J Surg 83:87
2. Henry GF, Defechereux T, Gramatica L et al (1999) Minimally invasive videoscopic parathyroidectomy by lateral approach. Arch Surg 384:298-301
3. Shimizu K, Akira S, Jasmi AY et al (1999) Video-assisted neck surgery: endoscopic resection of thyroid tumors with a very minimal neck wound. J Am Coll Surg 188:697-703
4. Ikeda Y, Takami H, Sasaki Y et al (2000) Endoscopic neck surgery by the axillary approach. J Am Coll Surg 191:336-340
5. Ohgami M, Ishii S, Ohmori T et al (2000) Scarless endoscopic thyroidectomy: breast approach better cosmesis. Surg Laparosc Endosc Percutan Tech 10:1-4
6. Miccoli P, Cecchini G, Conte M et al (1997) Minimally invasive, video-assisted parathyroid surgery for primary hyperparathyroidism. J Endocrinol Invest 20:429-430
7. Miccoli P, Bellantone R, Mourad M et al (2002) Minimally invasive video assisted thyroidectomy: a multi-institutional experience. World J Surg 26:972–975
8. Kim J, Giuliano AE, Turner RR et al (2006) Lymphatic mapping establishes the role of BRAF gene mutation in papillary thyroid carcinoma. Ann Surg 244-799-804
9. Pelizzo MR, Merante Boschin I, Toniato A et al (2006) Sentinel node mapping and biopsy in thyroid cancer: a surgical perspective. Biomed Pharmacother 60:405-408
10. Carcoforo P, Feggi L, Trasforini G et al (2007) Use of preoperative lymphoscintigraphy and intraoperative gamma-probe detection for identification of the sentinel lymph node in patients with papillary thyroid carcinoma. Eur J Surg Oncol 33:1075-1080

11. Wang J, Deng X, Jin X et al (2007) Management of the sentinel lymph node of papillary thyroid carcinoma in surgery. Lin Chung Er Bi Yan Hou Tou Jing Wai Ke Za Zhi 21(12): 543-547

12. Tükenmez M, Erbil Y, Barbaros U et al (2007) Radio-guided nonpalpable metastatic lymph node localization in patients with recurrent thyroid cancer. J Surg Oncol 96:534–538

13. Young-Sun K, Hyunchul R, Kyung T et al (2006) Radiofrequency ablation of benign cold thyroid nodules: initial clinical experience. Thyroid 16:361–367

14. Baek JH, Jehong HI, Kim YS et al (2008) Radiofrequency ablation for an autonomously functioning thyroid nodule. Thyroid 18:675–676

15. Pacella CM, Bizzarri G, Spiezia S et al (2004) Thyroid tissue: US-guided percutaneous laser thermal ablation. Radiology 232:272–280

16. Papini E, Bizzarri G, Pacella CM (2008) Percutaneous laser ablation of benign and malignant thyroid nodules. Curr Opin Endocrinol Diabetes Obes 15:434–439

17. Catalano MG, Costantino L, Fortunati N et al (2007) High energy shock waves activate 50-aminolevulinic acid and increase permeability to paclitaxel: antitumor effects of a new combined treatment on anaplastic thyroid cancer cells. Thyroid 17: 91–99

18. Fortunati N, Catalano MG, Arena K et al (2004) Valproic acid induces the expression of the Na+/I- symporter and iodine uptake in poorly differentiated thyroid cancer cells. J Clin Endocrinol Metab 89:1006–1009

19. Marchion DC, Bicaku E, Daud AI et al (2004) Sequence-specific potentiation of topoisomerase II inhibitors by the histone deacetylase inhibitor suberoylanilide hydroxamic acid. J Cell Biochem 92:223–237

20. Catalano MG, Fortunati N, Pugliese M et al (2005) Valproic acid induces apoptosis and cell cycle arrest in poorly differentiated thyroid cancer cells. J Clin Endocrinol Metab 90:1383–1389

21. Lo Gerfo P (1999) Bilateral neck exploration for parathyroidectomy under local anesthesia: a viable technique for patients with coexisting thyroid disease with or without sestamibi scanning. Surgery 126:1011–1014

22. Brunaud L, Ayav A, Zarnegar R et al (2008) Prospective evaluation of 100 robotic-assisted unilateral adrenalectomies. Surgery 144:995–1001

23. Adams S, Baum RP, Hertel A et al (1998) Intraoperative gamma probe detection of neuroendocrine tumors. J Nucl Med 39:1155–1160

24. Van Haren RM, Fitzgerald TR (2008) Intraoperative hand held gamma probe detection of a recurrent nonfunctional neuroendocrine tumor. JOP J Pancreas (Online) 9:704–707

25. Pelaez N, Busquets J, Ortega M et al (2005) Intraoperative gamma probe detection of lymph node recurrence of insulinomas. J Surg Oncol 91:209–211

Robots in Oncological Surgery

7

M. Morino, F. Rebecchi, L. Repetto

Introduction

The Robot Institute of America defines a robot as "an automatically controlled, reprogrammable, multipurpose, manipulator programmable in three or more axes, which may be either fixed in place or mobile for use in industrial automation applications" [1].

The term "robotic surgery" refers to the surgical technology that places a computer-assisted electro-mechanical instrument between the surgeon and the patient [2]. The exact term for the instruments currently used is "remote presence manipulator", since the available technology does not generally work without the explicit and direct control of a human operator. The key elements of this "remote presence" are the implementation of the surgeon's skills and the alteration of the traditional direct contact between surgeon and patient [3].

History

The term robot comes from the Czech *robota*, servant. It was used for the first time by the playwright Karel Capek in his drama "Rossum's Universal Robots" in 1921, and later at the beginning of the 1940s by Isaac Asimov in his short story entitled "Runaround".

Later on, robots entered the collective imagination thanks to the broad range of science fiction literature and the increasing, but not always positive, role played in movies. The shift from the fantasy to reality dates back to 1958, when General Motors introduced *Unimate* into the car manufacturing industry [4]. The introduc-

M. Morino (✉)
Centre of Mini-Invasive Surgery, S. Giovanni Battista University Hospital, Turin, Italy

New Technologies in Surgical Oncology. Antonio Mussa (Ed.)
© Springer-Verlag Italia 2010

tion of robotic technology into surgery is much more recent, having occurred over the past twenty years, encouraged by the progress of biomedical technology, particularly in the endoscopic technology field, and by the extensive development of information technology.

Robotic surgery was used for the first time in neurosurgery; it dates back to the first half the 1980s when the Unimate Puma 2000 was built specifically to be used with neurosurgical instruments in stereotactic biopsies [5]. Subsequently used in orthopedics (the introduction of Robodoc for hip replacement surgery dates back to 1992), robotic systems have been more recently used in general and specialized abdominal surgery. Computer Motion and Intuitive Surgical were the main manufacturers of robotic surgery systems until 2003, when Intuitive Surgical bought out Computer Motion.

Computer Motion was founded in 1989 by Yulun Wang. It marketed AESOP, which became the first surgical robot approved by the FDA (in 1994) and started the concept of solo-surgery. The same happened with the Zeus Robotic Microsurgical System, introduced in 1998 and used in 2001 for the first experience of remote surgery on humans [6]. Intuitive Surgical was established in 1995 on the basis of the technological achievements of the Stanford Research Institute; it developed and marketed the Da Vinci Surgical System, the only surgical manipulator on the market in 2003.

Currently the Da Vinci system is approved by the FDA for several surgical procedures; an advanced model is on the market. The Da Vinci Surgical System is a robotic remote manipulator made of three different parts: the workstation, or operating console (master), the surgical cart (slave) and the vision system.

Operating Console

The operating console is a non-sterile workstation that is kept distant from the operating table; it has wheels for easy movement, a power cable for connection to the electricity main and three more cables for connection to the slave (Fig. 7.1).

The operating console consists of several different parts:
- The *viewing window*, an area of the operating station that includes a stereo viewer (fixed eyepiece through which the surgeon sees the 3D image), as well as head sensors that detect the presence of the surgeon's head
- Two *control panels*, one on the surgeon's right side, the user switch panel, with several buttons (System, Emergency Stop, Stand-By, Ready, etc.) to maneuver the surgical cart, and another, the User Interface Panel, to program the scale of movement, i.e., the degree of transformation of movements by the master into the much finer movements of the tips of the instruments
- Two *joysticks*, or *master-grips*, to control the instruments and move the camera, connected to the robotic arms of the surgical cart; they can follow the movements of the surgeon's hands in every direction and translate them into precise movements of the robotic arms and the instruments connected to them

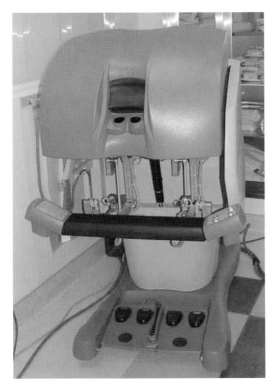

Fig. 7.1 Operator console (dimensions 166x97x158 cm, weight 227 kg)

- Five pedals or *foot switches* (coagulator, master alignment camera control, etc.)
- The *InSite^TM Vision System* is a sophisticated device incorporated into the Da Vinci that provides high-quality 3D vision of the surgical area. The InSite Vision system includes the 3D camera head, where the pictures acquired by the laparoscope through the separate optical channels are separately processed, 3D endoscopes that can be 0° or 30° and are fixed to the camera head during the operation, and the vision cart.

Surgical Cart

The surgical cart is located next to the operating table, partially inside the sterile area; its position changes depending on the surgical procedure (Fig. 7.2). It consists of a supporting column with:
- Two *instrument arms*: articulated systems connected to surgical instruments capable of precisely reproducing the movement performed by the surgeon at the console; the most recent model, the Da Vinci S, has three instrument arms
- A *camera arm*, central arm that controls the camera/endoscope group according to the movements made by the surgeon.

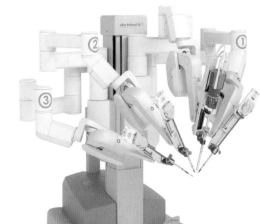

Fig. 7.2 Robotic arms (dimensions 198x94x97 cm, weight 544 kg)

Vision System

The system includes several devices that process and optimize the image quality during surgery.

The surgeon operates while seated at a console, his elbows resting on the support and his forehead positioned between two sensors that detect the presence of his head and act as a further control device. The surgeon's fingers grasp the master-grips connected by electro-mechanical devices to the robotic instruments. The central computer collects the input sent by the operator and transforms it into precise and fine movements by the camera and instruments.

The EndoWrist™ double articulation located at the tip of the instruments connected to the two robotic arms reproduces the six degrees of freedom typical of open surgery, as well as a gripping position, offering a total of seven degrees of freedom; the instruments can be articulated through 180° and rotated by 540°.

The instruments, which can be replaced during the operation, can be used a few times only and their use is automatically monitored and updated at the beginning of every procedure. Each instrument has a different life span (for instance, 18 procedures for the needle-holder, 10 for gripping instruments and scissors, 8 for the monopolar hook).

The Da Vinci system has several safety features. Each time the camera is moved and repositioned, the instruments stay still; the system automatically enters stand-by mode when the surgeon takes his head out of the console, and the instruments can be stopped during each positioning of the robotic arms. Furthermore, the entire system can be shut down immediately if necessary. The main limitations are the size and weight of the machine, which are unsuitable for the majority of operating rooms and make the machine difficult to maneuver; even the robotic arms are bulky and can collide with each other. Furthermore most instruments can be used only 10 times, increasing costs considerably [7,8] and they still do not come in the variety of shapes and sizes offered by conventional laparoscopic instruments. Technological innovation is likely provide solutions to these limitations in the near future.

Clinical Experiences in General Oncological Surgery

Robot-assisted Surgery in Esophageal Cancer

Esophagectomy is the only potentially curative strategy for the esophageal tumor with a cure rate of 10 to 50%. The mini-invasive approach was implemented in order to reduce the biological impact of esophagectomy and reduce post-operative pain. Less bleeding, shorter time in intensive care and a shorter overall hospital stay are important advantages of this type of approach, which also reduces post-operative morbidity and mortality with good results. However, some authors indicate it as being potentially "less oncological". This is probably due to the fact that, after the initial experience published by several authors, the limitations of the laparoscopic approach started to emerge. These mainly regard the learning curve in relation to a technique characterized by the difficult performance of the operating gestures in a very small space, using non-articulated instruments, with no tactile feedback and with 2D vision. The introduction of robotic technology can solve the aforementioned problems, since it offers the possibility of 3D vision, more freedom of the instruments and therefore more precision and sensitivity when manipulating tissues.

The literature describes two types of approach for the treatment of esophageal pathology with robotic technology: the transthoracic approach and the transhiatal approach. In both cases, the technique is similar to that used in traditional laparoscopic and laparotomic surgery.

Transthoracic Approach

The main problem of the classic thoracoscopy is that the movement of the instruments introduced into the intercostal spaces is limited by the ribs and therefore access to many thoracic areas is difficult and causes pain due to the "pressure" on the chest wall. Robotic surgery brilliantly solves this problem and thus constitutes an amazing progress. According to the data provided by the literature regarding this type of approach, there is a reduction in post-operative pain and therefore the use of painkillers, a better view and more accurate dissection of the paraesophageal tissues and lymph nodes. The limitations to this approach concern those patients that cannot tolerate unilateral ventilation for a long time, patients who suffer from pleural adhesions or have severe local invasion of the disease (larger than 4–5 cm in diameter), or those patients presenting mediastinal scar reactions from previous mediastinal surgery, infections or radiotherapy [9,10].

Transhiatal Approach

The number of patients treated with this technique is small; the literature tells us that this type of approach assures less bleeding, less cardio-pulmonary complications and is a possible alternative in the treatment of esophageal adenocarcinoma. The short period of follow-up and limited number of cases to date prevent judgment with regard to the long-term results from an oncological point of view [11–13].

The laparoscopic approach offers excellent vision for stomach immobilization and esophageal dissection up to the level of the lower pulmonary veins. The main advantages of this method are shorter operations, shorter time in intensive care and a shorter overall hospital stay. However mediastinal lymph-node dissection is difficult to perform with robots.

The thoracoscopic approach improves vision during esophageal mobilization and rear mediastinal lymph node dissection; it also facilitates esophageal dissection in the event of neoplasms in the mid and rear esophagus. However, the thoracoscopic approach is not free from disadvantages: first of all the patient needs to be repositioned in order to proceed with the operation after the thoracoscopic part; prolonged unilateral ventilation can expose the patient to serious pulmonary complications; access to the mediastinum is awkward if sufficient collapse of the lung is not obtained; and seeding of neoplastic cells may occur around the trocar. As a result this approach is not always recommended. A recent proposal to place the patient prone to avoid the need for selective intubation seems to have restored enthusiasm in the promoters of mini-invasive surgery.

The robotic technique with longer instruments and with 7 degrees of freedom results in operations performed in a very small space which overcome the limits found both in the laparoscopic and thoracoscopic techniques.

Robot-assisted Surgery in Stomach Cancer

The use of the robotic technique in the treatment of stomach cancer has been documented by very few authors, the first being Giulianotti in 2003 [14]. In Japan more than half of the distal gastrectomies for stomach cancers are performed via laparoscopy. This type of approach results in less postoperative pain and therefore less use of painkillers, a shorter hospital stay and an improvement in patient quality of life after laparoscopy in comparison with the laparotomic access. In the available literature, the use of robots seems to suggest easier performance of lymphadenectomies [13,14]. The advantages of this approach are mainly found in precise movements, the elimination of hand-tremors, 3D vision and the 7 degrees of freedom offered by robotic instruments. On the other hand the size of the equipment, the inadequacy in broad operating areas and the lack of tactile feedback make up the disadvantages of this approach, also pointed out in gastric oncological surgery. What emerges from the data presented in the literature is that the robotic approach to the surgical treatment of stomach cancer is feasible and its results are comparable to those of the traditional technique; the removal of lymph nodes for D2 lymphadenectomy is easy and safe [15,16]. As regards benefits in relation to the traditional laparoscopic technique, there are no differences in terms of hemorrhage, postoperative pain, use of painkillers, a return to eating and post-operative stay in comparison to the traditional laparoscopic technique.

Robot-assisted Surgery in Colorectal Cancer

Robotic technology provides advantages also for colorectal surgery, such as the stability of the camera, 3D vision, the ergonomics of the instruments, the elimination of tremors and the increased degrees of freedom resulting in the possibility of performing fine movements in small operating areas. In this sense the biggest contribution of robotic technology is not in colic surgery, where the laparoscopic operating area is quite wide, but in colorectal surgery, where it is very difficult to manipulate tissues in such a small operating area.

There are many studies which show the feasibility of colic and rectal resections using robotic technology, often in comparison to the classic laparoscopic technique; there are, however, no valid randomized trials with medium to long-term follow-up regarding oncological results [17,18].

Both right and left hemicolectomy are the same as for the traditional laparoscopic technique in terms of post-operative return to eating and mobilization. However, there are big differences regarding the operating time and cost of surgery [17–19]. The available literature shows that robotic surgery has important disadvantages, especially for right hemicolectomy, in terms of operating time and the difference in overall cost. These disadvantages are due mainly to the fact that the isoperistaltic ileocolic anastomosis is performed totally intra-abdominally with the aid of the robot. In contrast, in cases of right laparoscopic hemicolectomy, resection and anastomosis are performed after the exteriorization of the pertinent anatomical area. For left hemicolectomies there are differences regarding both the operating time and cost of surgery (higher in the case of robotic surgery), however these differences are not statistically significant. The literature provides no data regarding the "oncological" difference between the two types of approach. This is probably due to the fact that there is no difference between the techniques, but only between the ways of performing the standardized operating stages [20]. We can conclude that in the area of colic resections robotic technology supports the laparoscopic technique in terms of 3D vision and finer, more delicate manipulation and dissection of the structures, against higher costs and longer operating times, mainly with regard to operation on the right colon.

Anterior Resection of the Rectum

Anterior resection of the rectum is an interesting field of application for robotic surgery. Total mesorectal excision is the standard technique for surgical therapy of rectal tumors; the principle followed for this technique is the careful and precise dissection along the avascular plane that separates the presacral fascia from the mesorectal fascia. Robotic technology is a potential aid in this excision.

The robotic surgery technique in the anterior resection of the rectum can be compared to the laparoscopic technique. Despite there being no randomized trials with long-term follow-up, the data published in the literature do not reveal statistically important differences concerning the number of the lymph nodes removed, the distance of the lesion from the resection margin, bleeding and postoperative stay [21–24]. On the other hand, rectal surgery lacks tactile feedback, which is important to evaluate the tension of tissues at the moment of the dissection and in the event of simple traction with accidental lesions of the internal organs, and an increase in the cost of most of the work. Published data regarding the operating time varies, which seems to be connected to the training of the team and the nurses dedicated to the robotic activity.

Robots in Oncological Urology

Robots used in surgery improve the laparoscopic technique thanks to the aforementioned features. The precision of the gesture makes this instrument very effective each time reconstruction or demolition maneuvers are needed. These situations often occur in urology. When an organ affected by a neoplasm is removed, such as the bladder, prostate or part of a kidney, their continuity needs to be reconstructed with fine delicate sutures that require extreme precision. In urology, invasive techniques are very efficient, and it is in urology where robots are so useful.

Robots in the Treatment of Parenchymal Kidney Tumor

Given the bulky dimensions of the robotic arms, the aggression technique used in kidneys and the retroperitoneum can be performed exclusively with a transperitoneal approach, with the patient lying on the flank contralateral to the pathological kidney. The angle varies from 45° to 90°, according to operator preference.

Tumorectomy

Tumorectomy is the removal of the kidney lesion including a margin of at least 5 mm of healthy tissue. Operating robots can be of tremendous assistance in this setting. Most surgeons believe that the preparation of the kidney vessels is very important in the event of hemorrhage. Those of us who work with kidney transplants with donations from living donors are very attentive and sensitive to hot ischemia applied to the renal artery to overcome hemorrhages which occur in the area of the parenchymal incision. We agree with those authors who find it useful not to exceed twenty minutes of hot ischemia and believe that the robot could accelerate the parenchyma suture procedure after removal of the tumor. The duration of the hot ischemia can be reduced by applying argon-based coagulants or fibrin-based glues to the section of the renal parenchyma; these products are available on the market with different characteristics [25]. Undoubtedly the suture is easier, quicker and safe.

Partial Nephrectomy

Partial nephrectomy is the removal of the tumoral lesion including a margin at least 5 mm of healthy tissue. If the removal also includes part of the calyx and therefore the opening of the kidney outlets, the procedure is known as partial nephrectomy and not tumorectomy. In this case most surgeons not only believe that preparation of the renal vessels is useful, they actually consider it essential. The suture procedure for the calyx and sectioned kidney parenchyma takes longer. The suture must have an ischemic effect and must also seal the outlets [26–28]. The fourth passive arm is also very useful in this case. The easy opening and closure of the arm on the vessel that needs to be clamped enables the identification of severe bleeding and consequent application of new sutures.

Radical Nephrectomy and Enlarged Nephrectomy

Many authors, ourselves included, suggest that the cure of renal neoplasms lies in laparoscopy for a series of reasons which are now widely accepted. In this case, the limitations of operating robots are clear. The working area is smaller than a normal laparoscopic area [25–27]. The arms, especially when there are four of them, cannot perform extensive vertical or horizontal movements. The arms collide and get in the way of each other. The isolation of the upper pole might be difficult. Moreover, the robotic instruments do not come in as wide a range as those used in laparoscopy.

Robots and Bladder Cancer

Robotic surgical systems have improved the options of mini-invasive surgery. Performing a laparoscopic cystectomy with a robot is definitely a rather codified procedure with clear safety paths. The type of reconstruction is connected to the degree and type of invasion of the bladder tumor; furthermore, the habits of the surgeon play a very important role. Deciding whether or not to create an orthotopic neo-bladder or a urinary duct is a procedure which depends on many variables. In any case, using a robot can assure a fast and safe surgical path while maintaining the mini-invasive characteristics. Local relapses after the use of mini-invasive techniques, with considerably positive percentages, have suggested greater prudence also to operators with proven robotic skills. The procedure performed with a four-armed robot allows the surgeon, oncologist or urologist to operate without cutting too much. Robotics allows better control over vital and delicate nerves as well as more respect for muscle tissues, and facilitates fast recovery, reduces complications and makes the hospital stay shorter. In order to obtain good results in the treatment of bladder lesions, especially with robotic and surgical therapy, an early diagnosis is necessary [29,30].

Robotic Radical Prostatectomy

Currently the most efficient treatment for localized prostate cancer is surgery. Young patients are increasingly being diagnosed with prostate cancer, often localized. Surgery is the treatment which provides the greatest oncological reliability, especially in these cases. However, precisely due to their young age, the side effects of this treatment in these patients can have the greatest impact on quality of life, with particular regard to impotence and incontinence [31–33]. Besides the various surgical accesses to the prostatic gland (retropubic, perineal, transcoccygeal), recently the laparoscopic or robotic approach (transperitoneal or extraperitoneal) has also been added. The retropubic approach is still the most popular, since it allows the simultaneous removal of the pelvic lymph-nodes if necessary. Robotic laparoscopic prostatectomy is a procedure that combines laparoscopic skills with open surgery. Only in a few cases is it necessary to transform the laparoscopic procedure into traditional surgery, however the surgeon must be ready for anything. Scientific observation has confirmed that the perineal approach is the least used, despite being the first approach used. The small operative area and the surgeon's habits mean that this approach is either loved or hated by surgeons. Furthermore, recent studies have failed to confirm that the perineal approach can result in a higher number of positive surgical margins, as stated in other observations. There is a favorable attitude towards robots applied to the treatment of kidney tumor especially in the application of the kidney-sparing techniques. The same positive or cautiously positive attitude applies to cystectomy and subsequent reconstruction to restore continuity. There is a more critical attitude towards radical prostatectomy, both laparoscopic and robotic. Not everyone shares the same enthusiasm about mini-invasive techniques. Retropubic prostatectomy can be performed using either the transperitoneal or extraperitoneal method. These are the classic accesses which use safe and tested approaches. When carried out very carefully they are no more invalidating than modern techniques, nor do they provoke serious hemorrhages or side effects. Some detailed analyses suggest that open surgery techniques provide better oncological results than mini-invasive techniques. Furthermore, using magnifying glasses allows equally good vision of the anatomical structures in the surgical field as in laparoscopic or robotic techniques [31,32]. Lastly, it should be borne in mind that the perineal approach is the shortest surgical access for reaching the prostate.

References

1. Bann S, Khan M, Hernandez J et al (2003) Robotics in surgery. Am Coll Surg 5:784–795
2. Ballantyne GH (2002) Robotic surgery, telerobotic surgery, telepresence, and telementoring. Review of early clinical results. Surg Endosc 16:1389–1402
3. Herron DM, Marohn M (2008) A consensus document on robotic surgery. Surg Endosc 22:313–325
4. Hockstein NG, Gourin CG, Faust RA et al (2007) A history of robots: from science fiction to surgical robotics. J Robotic Surg 1:113–118

5. Kwoh YS, Hou J, Jonckheere EA et al (1988) A robot with improved absolute positioning accuracy for CT guided stereotactic brain surgery. IEEE Trans Biomed Eng 35:153–160

6. Wang Y, Sackier JM (1994) Robotically assisted laparoscopic surgery. From concept to development. Surg Endosc 8:63–66

7. Morino M, Benincà G, Giraudo G et al (2004) Robot assisted vs laparoscopic adrenalectomy: a prospective randomized controlled trial. Surg Endosc 18:1742–1746

8. Morino M, Pellegrino L, Giaccone C et al (2006) Randomized clinical trial of robot-assisted versus laparoscopic Nissen fundoplication. Br J Surg 93:553–558

9. Van Hillegersberg R, Boone J, Draaisma WA et al (2006) First experience with robot-assisted thoracoscopic esophagolymphadenectomy for esophageal cancer. Surg Endosc 20:1435–1439

10. Kernstine KH, DeArmond DT, Shamoun DM, Campos JH (2007) The first series of completely robotic esophagectomies with three-field lymphadenectomy: initial experience. Surg Endosc 21:2285–2292

11. Galvani CA, Gorodner MV, Moser F et al (2008) Robotically assisted laparoscopic transhiatal esophagectomy. Surg Endosc 22:188–195

12. Bodner JC, Zitt M, Ott H et al (2005) Robotic-assisted thoracoscopic surgery (RATS) for benign and malignant esophageal tumors. Ann Thorac Surg 80:1202–1206

13. Boone J, Borel Rinkes IHM, van Hillegersberg R (2008) Transhiatal robot-assisted esophagectomy. Surg Endosc 22:1139–1140

14. Giulianotti PC, Coratti A, Angelini M et al (2003) Robotics in general surgery. Arch Surg 138:777–784

15. Pugliese R, Maggioni D, Sanson F et al (2008) Robot-assisted laparoscopic gastrectomy with D2 dissection for adenocarcinoma: initial experience with 17 patients. J Robotic Surg 2:217–222

16. Anderson C, Ellenhorn J, Hellan M, Pigazzi A (2007) Pilot series of robot-assisted laparoscopic subtotal gastrectomy with extended lymphadenectomy for gastric cancer. Surg Endosc 21:1662–1666

17. Rawlings AL, Woodland JH, Vegunta RK, Crawford DL (2007) Robotic versus laparoscopic colectomy. Surg Endosc 21:1701–1708

18. Delaney CP, Lynch AC, Senagore AJ, Fazio VW (2003) Comparison of robotically performed and traditional laparoscopic colorectal surgery. Dis Colon Rectum 46:1633–1639

19. Huettner F, Rawlings AL, McVay WB, Crawford DL (2008) Robot-assisted laparoscopic colectomy: 70 cases–one surgeon. J Robotic Surg 2:227–234

20. Baik SH (2008) Robotic colorectal surgery. Yonsei Med J 49:891–896

21. Baik SH, Kang CM, Lee WJ et al (2007) Robotic total mesorectal excision for the treatment of rectal cancer. J Robotic Surg 1:99–102

22. Pigazzi A, Ellenhorn DI, Ballantyne GH, Paz B (2006) Robotic-assisted laparoscopic low anterior resection with total mesorectal excision for rectal cancer. Surg Endosc 20:1521–1525

23. Hellan M, Anderson C, Ellenhorn JDI et al (2007) Short-term outcomes after robotic-assisted total mesorectal excision for rectal cancer. Ann Surg Oncol 14:3168–3173

24. Baik SH (2008) Robotic total mesorectal excision for rectal cancer: it may improve survival as well as quality of life. Surg Endosc 22:1556

25. Breda A, Stepanian SV, Lam JS et al (2007) Use of haemostatic agents and glues during laparoscopic partial nephrectomy: a multi-institutional survey from the United States and Europe of 1347 cases. Eur Urol 52:798–803

26. Hyams ES, Kanofsky JA, Stifelman MD (2008) Laparoscopic Doppler technology: applications in laparoscopic pyeloplasty and radical and partial nephrectomy. Urology 71:952–956

27. Berger AD, Kanofsky JA, O'Malley RL et al (2008) Transperitoneal laparoscopic radical nephrectomy for large (more than 7 cm) renal masses. Urology 71:421–424

28. Figenshau R, Bhayani S, Venkatesh R, Wang A (2008) Robotic renal hilar control and robotic clip placement for partial nephrectomy. J Endourol 22:2657–2659

29. Chester JD, Hall GD, Forster M et al (2004) Systemic chemotherapy for patients with bladder cancer – current controversies and future directions. Cancer Treat Rev 30:343–358

30. Glas AS, Roos D, Deutekom M et al (2003) Tumor markers in the diagnosis of primary bladder cancer. A systematic review. J Urol 69:1775–1782

31. Ficarra V, Novara G, Artibani W et al (2009) Retropubic, laparoscopic, and robot-assisted radical prostatectomy: a systematic review and cumulative analysis of comparative studies. Eur Urol Jan 25 [Epub ahead of print]

32. Nielsen ME, Schaeffer EM, Marschke P, Walsh PC (2008) High anterior release of the levator fascia improves sexual function following open radical retropubic prostatectomy. J Urol 180:2557–2564

33. Patel VR, Palmer KJ, Coughlin G, Samavedi S (2008) Robot-assisted laparoscopic radical prostatectomy: perioperative outcomes of 1500 cases. J Endourol 22:2299–2305

Endoscopy and Surgical Oncology

8

C. De Angelis, A. Repici, M. Goss

Endoscopic therapy has emerged as a highly effective and minimally invasive way to control and cure early neoplasia of the digestive tract. Polypectomy has been a major advance, and most recently ablation and endoscopic mucosal resection seem to be highly successful in treating flat neoplastic areas involving the gut mucosa. The use of endoscopic ultrasonography (EUS) has resulted in improved accuracy for cancer staging, and EUS-guided fine-needle aspiration has been successful in obtaining tissue diagnosis outside the gut lumen. In advanced cancer, usually managed by multidisciplinary teams of oncologists, surgeons, and radiologists, the gastrointestinal endoscopist (GI) has assumed a key role not only in diagnosis but in palliation with the use of stents to bridge GI obstruction, ablation and the placement of tubes for drainage and feeding.

Local Treatment of GI Neoplasia: Endoscopic Mucosal Resection and Endoscopic Submucosal Dissection

Endoscopic Mucosal Resection

Endoscopic mucosal resection (EMR) has rapidly become a therapeutic modality that provides a valid alternative to surgical resection for the treatment of early cancers of the GI tract. By excision through the middle or deeper part of the submucosa, EMR allows complete and curative removal of areas of affected mucosa.

Submucosal injection used to facilitate EMR can help in the decision of whether or not to continue with the procedure, by the observation of a bleb formation with elevation of the overlying mucosa indicating the absence of deep submucosal involvement and the feasibility of EMR [1]. On the other hand, the dense fibrosis

C. De Angelis (✉)
Echoendoscopy Service and GEP Neuroendocrine Tumors Center, Department of Gastro Hepatology, S. Giovanni Battista University Hospital, Turin, Italy

8

associated with deep submucosal invasion prevents fluid infiltration through the submucosal connective tissue, decreasing bleb formation and elevation of the lesion. This so-called "non-lifting sign" has been found to have 100% sensitivity, 99% specificity, and 83% positive predictive value for invasive carcinoma in patients with early cancer of the colon [2]. Depth of tumor invasion can be precisely established by histological analysis of EMR specimens, which is part of the diagnostic algorithm for the evaluation of early gastric cancer [3] and, as recently suggested, for high-grade dysplasia and early adenocarcinoma arising in Barrett's esophagus.

EMR techniques can be separated into two major groups:

- "Lift-and-cut" method: lifting of the mucosal lesion is obtained by submucosal injection of a solution with the creation of a submucosal bleb that is strangulated by a snare and resected using electric cutting current. To maintain the fluid injection at the site of resection and render the procedure even safer than when saline alone is injected, the addition of epinephrine to decrease bleeding and the use of hypertonic saline, a 50% dextrose solution, or sodium hyaluronate to enhance formation and duration of a good bulge have been described. Indigo carmine is often added to the injectant to provide blue-green colour to the expanded submucosa to help in the assessment of depth during and after resection. Large lesions typically require piecemeal resection if possible performed during a single session [4]
- "Inject-suck-and-cut" method: Always after submucosal injection the lesion is aspirated and separated from the muscular coat and is resected by simple suction with a monofilament snare using different techniques (most commonly using a transparent plastic cap).

Assessment of endoscopic appearance is the initial step in suspecting advanced disease. Endoscopic resection should be done with curative intent. The existence of deep submucosally invasive cancer has a greater likelihood of regional lymph-node metastases and these are best addressed surgically. The technique of piecemeal removal may hinder the pathologist's ability to interpret the depth of invasion unless collected specimens are well oriented. More advanced disease can be judged endoscopically by the configuration of the lesion, mucosal pit pattern, non-lifting of the lesion with submucosal injection, and the use of endoscopic ultrasound (EUS) for staging. The appearance of ulceration, central depression, nodularity, and bowel-wall deformity is generally associated with advanced cancer; however, this is subject to interobserver variability. Magnifying colonoscopy with chromoendoscopy may be advantageous with detailed pit pattern analysis to predict the presence of cancer and its depth of invasion. EUS is widely available and has been well investigated. For superficial colonic lesions, a high frequency (12–20 MHz) probe can be used throughout the length of the colon and higher-quality images obtained. Early reports of 88% accuracy in determining depth of invasion by EUS have been tempered in later series (37–66%). The depth of invasion was staged in six categories (mucosa, submucosa 1–3, muscularis propria 1 and 2). If the depth of invasion is grouped into only two categories (mucosa with submucosa 1 and submucosa 2 with muscularis propria) to determine clinically relevant information such as the applicability of endoscopic mucosal resection (EMR), the accuracy of depth of invasion improves to 86–88.9%.

EMR in the Esophagus

The indications for EMR in the treatment of esophageal cancer are not well established. The available surgical experience suggests that the risk of lymph node metastasis increases with depth of invasion. Lymph node metastases have been reported to occur in 0 to 33% of patients with adenocarcinoma limited to the mucosa [5]. This risk increases to up to 50% when submucosal invasion occurs. Based on the available evidence, EMR should be performed for lesions shown to be confined to the mucosa.

EMR in the Stomach

The risk of lymph node metastasis in gastric adenocarcinoma increases with the depth of tumor penetration. Lesions confined to the mucosa are associated with a lower risk of lymph node involvement (0 to 3%), which increases to 20% for tumors extending deep in the submucosa [6]. Japanese investigators have determined that the diameter of the tumor, lymphatic involvement, depth of submucosal invasion, and extent of horizontal cancerous submucosal involvement significantly correlates with nodal involvement [7]. Absolute indications for gastric EMR include well- or moderately differentiated type IIa/IIb adenocarcinoma (the slightly elevated flat type) smaller than 2 cm or type IIc (slightly depressed type) without ulcer formation smaller than 1 cm. Lymph node metastasis is found in only 0.01% of such cases, and prognosis after this treatment is comparable to that of surgical resection for early gastric cancer in completely resected cases [8]. For type IIc undifferentiated early gastric cancer, a consensus has not been reached. Relative indications include (1) well-differentiated mucosal cancer < 30 mm in size without ulcer or ulcer scar, (2) well-differentiated mucosal cancer 20 mm in size with ulcer or ulcer scar, (3) poorly differentiated cancer <10 mm in size, and (4) sm 1 cancer <20 mm in size without ulcer or ulcer scars. Recurrence after histopathologically documented eradication was observed in 1.9% of the patients.

EMR in the Colon

Flat (non-polypoid) lesions larger than 1 cm are classified as the lateral spreading type or lateral spreading tumor. This is further classified into the flat type and granular (or nodular aggregate) type. The incidence of cancer with submucosal invasion appears to be higher in flat-type lateral spreading tumors. Endoscopic findings with statistical significance are presence of depression, large (>10 mm) nodule, uneven nodularity, and a size greater than 30 mm compared with less than 20 mm in addition to histological type. The rate of malignancy in these large lesions has been reported to be 5–15% [9]. In a large single-centre study, the rate of malignancy was 10.4% for lesions of 16–20 mm and 22.1% for lesions of greater than 20 mm, thus suggesting the larger the size of the lesion, the more likely it is to harbor invasive cancer. The endoscopic treatment for large lesions essentially is snare polypectomy. The large lesions of the protruded type can be treated by ordinary snare-and-cut polypectomy. It is difficult to snare the large lesions that are sessile or flat and adequate resection margins cannot always be obtained. Thus endoscopic treatment has been mostly done with a resection using piecemeal technique (endoscopic piecemeal mucosal resection) with or without submucosal saline injection. The benefit of the saline injection technique has not been evaluated in direct comparison with the no-saline-injection technique, but it is easy to speculate that it allows more tissue to be snared with lower risk of perforation since saline injection separates the submucosal layer from the muscularis propria.

The major drawback of piecemeal polypectomy is the impairment of complete histopathological evaluation of the resected lesion which is critical in predicting patient outcome. Therefore, en bloc resection of the lesion should always be attempted when possible, and subsequent complete removal can be achieved with piecemeal resection as needed.

Additional treatment with argon plasma coagulation (APC) has been used to obtain complete eradication of neoplastic tissue after piecemeal polypectomy. APC treatment was reported to reduce the adenoma recurrence regardless of whether the piecemeal polypectomy is complete or incomplete. The use of APC is rather easy, yet effective in eradicating residual adenoma after incomplete piecemeal resection when further polypectomy cannot be performed. Resected margins must be carefully evaluated to assess the completeness of the resection. Magnification chromoendoscopy could improve the effectiveness of complete endoscopic resection. Unluckily, magnification chromoendoscopy is currently limited in availability and by the need for endoscopist training.

EMR in the Duodenum

There is a limited number of studies evaluating the role of EMR in the treatment of duodenal lesions. Benign and malignant tumors of the papilla of Vater are a growing indication for duodenal EMR [10]. Long-term success rates ranging from 70% to 80% have been reported. When a papillary lesion has been resected endoscopically, surveillance duodenoscopy is mandatory because recurrent disease occurs in up to one fourth of cases [11], although most recurrences have been treated successfully using endoscopic methods. Also EUS can be useful in the follow-up.

EMR complications

- Bleeding: the most frequent complication of EMR, which has been reported to occur in 1.5 to 24% of cases
- Perforation: the most worrisome complication. It is uncommon with EMR techniques. Perforation occurs when the muscle layer is included in the snare resection. Generally this is due to a lack of submucosal saline solution injection while performing the procedure
- Stenosis: especially as a consequence of EMR in the esophagus with deep thermal injury of the esophageal wall.

Endoscopic Submucosal Dissection

A newly developed technique is endoscopic submucosal dissection (ESD) which requires the use of special knives. This technique is suitable for en bloc resection of large lesions in the gastrointestinal tract which otherwise would be resected in piece-meal fashion. It was developed for large gastric lesions and is now being used in other locations. Perforation rates were initially high but have subsequently improved. In the hands of an expert, the rates of bleeding and perforation were lower than 1%.

For the curative treatment of mucosal colonic lesions, the most important issue is the completeness of the resection. This task can be difficult to achieve in large ses-sile polyps and residual tumor may be left behind, leading to local recurrence. Conventional techniques of EMR are thought to be inadequate for en bloc resection of large colonic lesions. The multiple fragments that result from this piecemeal resection make the histopathological evaluation of the completeness of polyp removal difficult. Therefore, en bloc resection with a satisfactory tumor cell-negative margin is considered a more desirable outcome. The technical limitations in endo-scopic treatment of large colonic lesions can sometimes be overcome by a device enabling the performance of en bloc resection, thus allowing the acquisition of a sin-gle large specimen for the correct evaluation of the resection margins.

In 1995, Hosokawa and Yoshida developed a new device for EMR: the insulated-tip electrosurgical knife (It-knife), which has a ceramic bulb at the tip to prevent injury to deeper layers of the GI tract. EMR with an It-knife made possible en bloc resections of large early stage gastric cancers with a reduction in the recurrence rate. Subsequently, a number of different knives with specific technical peculiarities, like the hook-knife or the flex-knife, have been introduced in clinical practice by Japanese endoscopists with large experience in submucosal dissection of early gastric cancer.

As for standard colonic EMR, formation of a good submucosal cushion under the targeted mucosa is one of the most important elements for successful ESD. By mix-ing a small amount of indigo carmine dye or methylene blue into the injected solu-tion, the target area can be distinguished much more easily from the non-injected area even after pre-injections of normal saline. After a sufficient lifting of the lesion is produced, a small mucosal incision with a needle knife is created in the two oppo-site areas of the tumor and thereafter the circumferential mucosal incision with a knife can be performed safely. A cylindrical transparent hood, 8 mm in length or a standard transparent cap, attached to the endoscope tip also are very helpful for the safety of mucosal incision by reducing unintentional movements of the colonic wall towards the needle knife. However, this technique is more demanding and only spo-radically used for resection of non-gastric lesions such as large colonic neoplasms.

As for gastric ESD, endoscope retroflexion in the colon is one of the most required maneuvers to approach large lesions, especially those located behind folds on the proximal end of tight turns or involving more than 2/3 of circumference. In order to facilitate retroflexion, in particular in the left colon, it is possible to use a therapeutic gastroscope whose flexibility is greater than a standard colonoscope and allows an easy retroflexion in all the colonic segments. The procedure is progressive-ly performed by advancing the ESD while sliding the tip of the endoscope with a hood under the dissected mucosa. Effective control of bleeding during the procedure is a priority. This complication must be promptly controlled whenever it occurs, regardless of its severity. An endoscopic field which is dirty with fresh blood or clots makes it difficult to identify the submucosal resection plane as well as the lesion margin. Blood vessels can be recognized during the submucosal incision, at this moment, the output mode is changed to the APC mode. Because the voltage of the latter is higher than the coagulation mode, small blood vessels can be cut without bleeding. Hemorrhage can also be prevented or stopped by using hemostatic forceps.

Perforation is a major concern as a possible complication of ESD. This event can be minimized by sufficiently thickening the submucosa by proper injection of sodium hyaluronate and careful selection of the layer for incision. The causes determining the risk of wall perforation include the reduced room of colonic lumen and the variety of angles and folds that make the proper control of knife movements very difficult as it may prove challenging to control both the depth and the direction of the cut at the same time. The risk can be further increased when the lesion is infiltrating the submucosa and injection cannot adequately create a submucosal cushion. For this reason, careful inspection of the submucosal layer during the dissection is required to identify submucosal tissue or irregularities compatible with deep neoplastic invasion. When a perforation is made during the procedure, it is usually small and recognized immediately; therefore, it can be closed with endoscopic clip placements and can be managed conservatively.

Endoluminal Palliation

New techniques have expanded the role of endoscopy in the diagnosis, staging, therapy, and palliation of malignancies. Self-expanding metal stents (SEMS) have been used as an alternative to surgery in the palliation of luminal obstruction due to GI cancer. The major sites of use include the esophagus, the gastroduodenum, and the colon. SEMS can be placed through the scope under fluoroscopic or endoscopic guidance [12]. Colorectal and gastroduodenal cancers make up a significant proportion of gastrointestinal malignancies. Intestinal obstruction is a common presentation of colorectal cancer, and is often seen in non-gastrointestinal cancers invading or metastasising to the gastrointestinal tract. Management of intestinal obstruction is challenging because the patients are often acutely ill and debilitated from underlying malignancy. Severe vomiting leading to electrolyte imbalance, sepsis, ischemia, and impending perforation are the well-known features of intestinal obstruction. Associated morbidity and mortality are high. Not surprisingly, acute colonic obstruction is considered a surgical emergency. A number of surgical and non-surgical modalities are available for treatment of malignant intestinal obstruction. Unfortunately, surgery is not a viable option for most patients with gastroduodenal malignancies: 40% of gastric cancer patients and 95% of pancreatic cancer patients with duodenal involvement are not candidates for curative resection. Surgical palliation can be achieved through gastroenterostomy or gastrojejunostomy. However, such surgical procedures carry a high morbidity rate in advanced cancer patients [13]. Gastroduodenal obstruction in non-surgical candidates is typically treated with nasogastric intubation or a 2-valve gastrojejunostomy tube, allowing for decompression and feeding. Other gastro-duodenal palliative techniques, such as endoluminal irradiation, laser ablation, and chemical injection, have somewhat limited application in the management of large exophytic tumors. None of the above-mentioned modalities allow for adequate oral food intake, and all are associated with significant patient discomfort.

Esophageal carcinoma affects a heterogeneous population. In the esophagus, the small diameter of the SEMS allows for easier deployment without aggressive dilation. A systematic review of the use of SEMS for gastroduodenal malignancies reviewed published data on 606 patients. Technical success in SEMS placement was achieved in 589 patients (97%). Functional relief of symptoms was achieved in 89% of the patients in whom the SEMS was deployed. Acute complications including bleeding and perfo-ration were reported in seven patients (1.2%). Long-term complications included stent obstruction mainly due to tumor in-growth (18%) and stent migration (5%). The medi-an survival was 12 weeks [14].

The use of SEMS in colorectal cancer is becoming more commonplace. It can be placed across an obstructing colonic mass for preoperative decompression or palliation [14]. The success rates for stent deployment and clinical decompression range from 70 to 95%. In addition to relief of colonic obstruction, preoperative stent placement allows for adequate staging of disease and bowel preparation before surgery. The ability to cleanse the bowel proximal to the obstruction may allow for a one-stage colonic resection without the need for diverting colostomy. In addition, preoperative chemoradiation is possible because the stent allows for decompression of the bowel and adequate nutrition during neo-adjuvant therapy [15]. In the case of an unresectable tumor, the SEMS can be left in place for relief of symptoms. Multiple studies suggest that endoscopic placement of SEMS is a safe and effective method to relieve luminal obstruction due to GI malignan-cies. Emerging issues in stent technology include the development of removable stents; drug-eluting stents; and improved stent design to optimize patency, reduce gastro-esophageal reflux, and minimize stent migration.

Removable stents are appealing for therapy of non-malignant strictures that do not respond to routine dilatation. Potential applications include anastomotic strictures and radiation strictures. Preliminary experience suggests that this device is effective and safe, but larger studies are needed [14]. New stent design and manufacturing methods have allowed development of anti-reflux stents and other custom stent shapes using laser etch-ing of solid metal tubes. These technologies have the capability of producing more precise shape and mechanical properties for difficult locations, such as the upper esophagus.

Narrow-Band Imaging Endoscopy for the Diagnosis of Malignant and Premalignant Gastrointestinal Lesions

Narrow-band imaging (NBI) is a novel endoscopic technique that may enhance the accuracy of diagnosis by using narrow-bandwidth filters in a red-green-blue (R/G/B) sequential illumination system [16]. This results in different images at distinct levels

8

of the mucosa and increases the contrast between the epithelial surface and the subjacent vascular pattern. It has been postulated that NBI may lead to the same contrast enhancement capabilities as chromoendoscopy, but without the toil of using dye agents [17,18]. Magnifying endoscopy by using NBI has two distinct applications: the analysis of the surface architecture of the epithelium (pit pattern) and the analysis of the vascular network [19]. NBI may demonstrate the disorganization of the pit pattern and vascular pattern of the gastrointestinal mucosa in inflammatory and neoplastic (premalignant and malignant) lesions of the esophagus, stomach and large bowel. The main usefulness of this technique is to identify and target biopsies in areas of intestinal metaplasia, dysplasia and carcinoma [20,21]. Endoscopic examination with NBI is carried out in the usual way; there are no special requirements for preparation and sedation of the patient, but additional information is obtained by analyzing the mucosal surface, including vascular pattern in greater detail [22]. Secondary prevention of cancer requires early detection at the stage when the lesion is still curable. Magnifying endoscopy by using NBI provides the most effective method of detecting premalignant and malignant precursors of advanced cancer in which the tumor process is restricted to the superficial layers of the gastrointestinal wall. Discrete epithelial premalignant lesions in mucosa of the digestive tract are the first step in the progression to superficial malignancy and then to advanced cancer. Premalignant lesions often develop against a background of inflammation and diffuse alterations in the mucosa; these are considered to be risk factors for cancer and are called "premalignant conditions". Premalignant conditions of the gastrointestinal tract include intestinal metaplasia of the esophagus and stomach, chronic gastritis associated with *H. pylori* infection, chronic inflammation in ulcerative colitis, and gastrointestinal adenomas [23].

Oncology and the Challenge of Endoscopic Ultrasound

Endoscopic ultrasound (EUS) has been one of the most important innovations to occur in GI endoscopy during the last 25 years. It has extended the range of possibilities for endoscopic diagnosis, supplying the endoscopist with the unequalled opportunity to see not only the mucosal surface but within and beyond the wall of the GI tract.

The technique combines the potentials of two methods, endoscopy and ultrasonography, by means of a small ultrasound transducer, which is fitted on the tip of a particular endoscope (echoendoscope). Lesions even as small as 1–2 mm can be visualized in the gastro-intestinal wall, the pancreas, the bile ducts and so forth.

The development during the late 1980s of small miniaturized echographic probes (miniprobes), capable of passing through the operating channel of normal endoscopes (gastroscopes and colonoscopes), has made it possible to apply the echoendoscopic technique during the course of a normal gastroscopy or colonoscopy, whenever the need occurs; it has also made it possible to pass through stenotic sections (namely with a lumen so narrow as to prevent the passage of any other instrument either endoscopic or echoendoscopic), to introduce the echoendoscopic probes into the cecum and into the distal ileum and above all its constantly greater miniaturization has made it possible to penetrate with the miniprobe inside the bile ducts and the pancreatic duct, for the diagnosis of pathological strictures or small calculi and tumors not visible with any other imaging method available today (echoendoscopy with intraductal miniprobe, i.e., IntraDuctal UltraSound, IDUS) [24,25].

At present, several therapeutic options are available in various oncologic diseases: in each tumor careful staging is essential for correct management. "Selection is the silent partner of success": staging has today a deep impact on treatment choices and an appropriate staging-oriented therapy improves patient prognosis and quality of life.

Today EUS is still the most accurate imaging technique for pre-therapeutic clinical staging, both T and N, of early GI neoplasia. However, conventional EUS, with dedicated echoendoscope (5, 7.5 and 12 MHz), has not sufficient accuracy in differentiating T1m from T1sm cancers [26]. Small miniaturized echographic probes (miniprobes), which can be passed through the operative channel of a standard endoscope, can achieve better results providing high spatial resolution of the GI wall, depicted as a 9-layered structure instead of a 5-layered one, seen with the lowest frequencies. Particularly these higher frequencies would allow the visualization of the muscularis mucosae, which is crucial in distinguishing intramucosal from submucosal lesions. Miniprobes can assist EMR and increase its safety by reducing the risk of complications, especially perforative ones [27].

The visualisation of a suspicious lymph node may suggest surgery or, in selected cases, EUS-guided fine needle aspiration (EUS-FNA) in order to confirm or exclude metastatic lymph node involvement. The introduction of EUS-FNA is a clear improvement in the accuracy of nodal staging of GI tract tumors.

One of the more relevant advantages of EUS compared with other imaging techniques, such as transabdominal US, CT and MRI is its superior pancreatic parenchymal resolution.

The results of EUS have been shown to be even better in small tumors, less than 3 or 2 cm, where sensitivity of US and CT decreased to only 29% [28]. However in the last ten years EUS has had to bear the weight of the rapidly evolving technology of radiological imaging modalities (Multidetector helical CT and MRI) and finally also the advent and the evolution of nuclear imaging such as positron emission tomography (PET) and the integrated approach PET/CT [29].

In this challenge EUS has been mainly supported by the advent of interventional EUS (EUS-FNA). In contrast to the very high sensitivity previously shown, specificity of EUS is limited, especially when inflammatory changes are present. The ability to perform EUS-FNA may overcome some of the specificity problems encountered with EUS in distinguishing benign from malignant lesions, allowing an improvement of EUS accuracy, mainly as a result of enhanced specificity, without losing too much in sensitivity [30].

Overall EUS is superior to CT for the detection of pancreatic cancer, for T staging and for vascular invasion of the spleno-portal confluence. The two tests appear to be equivalent for N staging, overall vascular invasion and assessment of resectability.

EUS-FNA has become the preferred modality for puncturing the pancreas [29,30].

8

References

1. Ishiguro A, Uno Y, Ishiguro Y et al (1999) Correlation of lifting versus non-lifting and microscopic depth of invasion in early colorectal cancer. Gastrointest Endosc 50:329–333
2. Uno Y, Munakata A (1994) The non-lifting sign of invasive colon cancer. Gastrointest Endosc 40:485–489
3. Tada M (2001) Endoscopic mucosal resection of the stomach: initial description. Gastrointest Endosc Clin N Am 11:499–510
4. Kanamori T, Itoh M, Yokoyama Y et al (1996) Injection-incision-assisted snare resection of large sessile colorectal polyps. Gastrointest Endosc 43:189–195
5. Clark G, Peters J, Ireland A et al (1994) Nodal metastasis and sites of recurrence after en bloc esophagectomy for adenocarcinoma. Ann Thorac Surg 58:646–653
6. Yamao T, Shirao K, Ono H et al (1996) Risk factors for lymph node metastasis from intramucosal gastric carcinoma. Cancer 77:602–606
7. Takekoshi T, Baba Y, Ota H et al (1994) Endoscopic resection of early gastric carcinoma: results of a retrospective analysis of 308 cases. Endoscopy 26:352–358
8. Makuuchi H, Kise Y, Shimada H et al (1999) Endoscopic mucosal resection for early gastric cancer. Semin Surg Oncol 17:108–116
9. Tanaka S, Haruma K, Oka S et al (2001) Clinicopathologic features and endoscopic treatment of superficially spreading colorectal neoplasms larger than 20 mm. Gastrointest Endosc 54:62–66
10. Kim MH, Lee SK, Seo DW et al (2001) Tumors of the major duodenal papilla. Gastrointest Endosc 54:609–620
11. Binmoeller KF, Boaventura S, Ramsperger K et al (1993) Endoscopic snare excision of benign adenomas of the papilla of Vater. Gastrointest Endosc 39:127–131
12. Dormann A, Meisner S, Verin N et al (2004) Self-expanding metal stents for gastroduodenal malignancies: systematic review of their clinical effectiveness. Endoscopy 36:543–550
13. Pungpapong S, Raimondo M, Wallace MB et al (2004) Problematic esophageal strictures: emerging indications for self-expandable silicone stents. Am J Gastroenterol 99:AB363
14. Baron TH (2001) Expandable metal stents for the treatment of cancerous obstruction of the gastrointestinal tract. N Engl J Med 344:1681–1687
15. Adler DG, Young-Fadok TM, Smyrk T et al (2002) Preoperative chemoradiation therapy after placement of a self-expanding metal stent in a patient with an obstructing rectal cancer: clinical and pathologic findings. Gastrointest Endosc 55:435–437
16. Tajiri H, Matsuda K, Fujisaki J (2002) What can we see with the endoscope? Present status and future perspectives. Dig Endosc 14:131–137
17. Kara MA, Peters FP, Rosmolen WD et al (2005) High-resolution endoscopy plus chromoendoscopy or narrow-band imaging in Barrett's esophagus: a prospective randomized crossover study. Endoscopy 37:929–936
18. Sambongi M, Igarashi M, Obi T et al (2000) Analysis of spectral reflectance of mucous membrane for endoscopic diagnosis. Med Phys 27:1396–1398
19. Kiesslich R, Jung M (2002) Magnification endoscopy: does it improve mucosal surface analysis for the diagnosis of gastrointestinal neoplasias? Endoscopy 34:819–822
20. Sharma P, Weston AP, Topalovski M et al (2003) Magnification chromoendoscopy for the detection of intestinal metaplasia and dysplasia in Barret's oesophagus. Gut 52:24–27
21. No authors listed (2005) Paris workshop on columnar metaplasia in the esophagus and the esophagogastric junction. Paris, France, December 11–12, 2004. Endoscopy 37:879–920
22. Kuznetsov K, Lambert R, Rey J-F (2006) Narrow-band imaging: potential and limitations. Endoscopy 38:76–81

23. Lambert R and the Endoscopic Classification Review Group (2005) Update on the Paris classification of superficial neoplastic lesions in the digestive tract. Endoscopy 37:570–578

24. Yasuda K, Mukai H, Nakajima M (1992) Clinical application of ultrasonic probes in the biliary and pancreatic duct. Endoscopy 24(Suppl 1):370–375

25. De Angelis C, Martini M, Repici A et al (2007) Instruments and accessories for diagnostic endoscopic ultrasound (radial scanning and miniprobes). Minerva Med 98:253–260

26. Hasegawa N, Niwa Y, Arisawa T et al (1996) Preoperative staging of superficial esophageal carcinoma: comparison of an ultrasound probe and standard endoscopic ultrasonography. Gastrointest Endosc 44:388–393

27. Waxman I, Saitoh Y, Raju GS et al (2002) High-frequency probe EUS-assisted endoscopic mucosal resection: a therapeutic strategy for submucosal tumors of the GI tract. Gastrointest Endosc 55:44–49

28. Yasuda K, Mukai H, Nakajima M (1995) Endoscopic ultrasonography diagnosis of pancreatic cancer. Gastrointest Endosc Clin N Am 5:699–712

29. De Angelis C, Repici A, Carucci P et al (2007) Pancreatic cancer imaging; the new role of endoscopic ultrasound. JOP 8(Suppl I):85–97

30. De Angelis C, Senore C, Ciccone G et al (2005) Accuracy of endoscopic ultrasound guided fine needle aspiration (FNA) in the diagnosis of solid pancreatic masses: a systematic review of the literature. Endoscopy 37(Suppl I):A282–283

Senologic Oncology and Reconstructive Surgery

9

S. Bruschi, P. Bogetti, R. Bussone

Historical Background

A century of breast cancer surgery has seen the evolution of a number of techniques for the surgical treatment of breast carcinoma by surgery. New knowledge of the natural history of breast carcinoma, the introduction of adjuvant therapies and increasingly early diagnosis have naturally led to a change in surgical treatment. The principal stages along this pathway have basically been three. First, the entity of surgical demolition has been reduced as well as the morbidity associated with it. From Halsted's radical mastectomy, through the variants proposed by Patey and Madden, we arrived at the removal of the glandular structure only, with dissection of axillary lymph nodes. Crile's studies in the sixties demonstrated the systemic nature of the disease, disproving Halsted's principle of en bloc removal of suspect tissue, and thus opening the door to conservative surgery [1].

The conservative surgery approach to breast carcinoma then became fully established thanks to the Milan randomized clinical trials of the seventies and eighties. The studies demonstrated that wide excision of the tumor plus radiotherapy (RT) obtained the same survival rates as with radical mastectomy and, moreover, that more limited excisions and the absence of radiotherapy produced the same rates of survival but greater rates of local recurrence.

Fisher's studies confirmed that the survival rate remained unchanged both after radical mastectomy and after varying degrees of wide excision with or without RT, while what changed was the rate of local recurrence. According to Fisher, local recurrence ought, however, to be considered an unfavorable prognostic index, there being no causality link between local recurrence and death from breast carcinoma [2].

It was seen that in 25% of cases local recurrence was the cause of death [3]. From this information it was deduced that between the two extremes, radical mastectomy on one side and conservative surgery + RT on the other, an intermediate route can be taken.

S. Bruschi (✉)
Plastic Surgery Unit, S. Giovanni Battista University Hospital, Turin, Italy

New Technologies in Surgical Oncology. Antonio Mussa (Ed.)
© Springer-Verlag Italia 2010

9

Even though conservative surgery is now practiced on large scale and accepted as a safe procedure, mastectomy still remains the treatment of choice for some patients. However, from the point of view of oncological safety and esthetic outcomes, the dichotomy "conservative therapy vs mastectomy" is now outdated and inappropriate, as the recent techniques, while safeguarding surgical radicality, have enabled increasingly better esthetic outcomes.

The sentinel lymph node biopsy proposed by Morton for melanoma and then extended to breast carcinoma constitutes the second important change in treatment for breast carcinoma. Axillary lymphadenectomy was the standard therapy for breast carcinoma for a long time, both because the histological status of axillary lymph nodes is the most important prognostic factor for survival, and so that regional control of the disease would be ensured. This procedure takes on therapeutic value in only one third of cases, while it has purely diagnostic significance in the remaining 70%, against a high rate of complications of around 50%. The principal complications include lymphedema, lymphangitis, phlebitis, pain, functional block and sensitive intercostobrachial nerve lesion.

The sentinel lymph node biopsy, introduced into clinical practice towards the end of the nineties, was validated by a number of clinical trials and two randomized clinical trials, and is today recognized as an accurate technique for evaluating lymph node involvement with very low morbidity [4].

The methods tested and validated for sentinel lymph node identification envisage the use of a vital dye with strong lymphotropism (Patent Blue-V), a radioactive tracer (99m Tc) or a combination of both. The experience of different authors demonstrates reliable detection rates varying from 65 to 90% for the vital dye and from 94 to 99% for the tracer [5,6]. It is common practice to use both methods, but in the case of choice, it is preferable to use the radioactive tracer; the results obtained justify the higher costs of this technique.

Although national and international guidelines have been published on the indications and modalities of performing the sentinel lymph node biopsy, the literature highlights considerable variability in the research and analysis technique. In the near future it will be necessary to bring the different methods to uniformity to then be able to compare the results of the different treatments.

The third consists in the evolution of RT techniques with the objective of reducing irradiation volume and contracting therapy times, as indicated by the abbreviation APBI, accelerated partial breast irradiation. The new techniques proposed include interstitial brachytherapy, mammosit, external band 3D RT and intraoperative radiotherapy (IORT).

Conservative Mastectomies

Skin Sparing Mastectomy

Introduced by Toth and Lappert in 1991, skin sparing mastectomy (SSM) constitutes the link between conservative surgery and modified or total radical mastectomy. It is able to ensure good local control of the disease with the minimum esthetic outcome, also enabling immediate breast reconstruction by expandable prosthesis. It provides for removal of the breast gland, the nipple–areola complex, scars of previous biopsies and the skin overlying the tumor, conserving as much as possible the cutaneous envelope and the inframammary fold.

From 1991 to 1999 numerous non-randomized clinical trials were conducted to compare the rate of local recurrence after SSM with that following conventional surgery and the literature necessary to confirm oncological safety was prolific [7–9].

The procedure is currently indicated with certainty for T1 tumors with an extended DICS component, multicentric T1 tumors, T2 tumors without possibility of conservative treatment, or following neoadjuvant chemotherapy, while it is contraindicated for locally advanced tumors, cutaneous involvement and patients who are smokers, diabetic or were previously irradiated, due to the risk of ischemic suffering of the cutaneous flap.

Based on the type of incision and the quantity of skin removed four types of SSM are singled out: type I for prophylactic mastectomies and non-palpable tumors; type II for superficial tumors or scars of previous biopsies close to the areola; type III if the tumor or previous scar is far from the areola; type IV, used in ptotic and large breasts combined with contralateral symmetrization. Over the course of the years some changes have been made to the technique proposed by Toth and Lappert regarding above all the type of incision. In type I SSM the periareolar incision with 'tobacco pouch' stitching has been described and, as a development of this, the star or comet incision [10]. This type of approach guarantees better healing by primary intention and consequently better esthetic outcomes. In type IV SSM, to obviate the frequent cutaneous necrosis at the point of conjunction of the T, Skoll proposed deepithelisation rather than removal of the area between the two vertical arms of the T and around 2 cm below the horizontal arm [11]. Our tendency is to use the "L" incision, with the aim of avoiding the complications linked with the "T" incision.

With regard to modified radical mastectomy or total mastectomy, since SSM conserves the cutaneous envelope and the inframammary fold it enables minimal scar outcomes to be obtained, but above all facilitates immediate reconstruction and reduces the need for symmetrization of the controlateral breast. On the other hand it is certainly a more complex technique that entails a greater risk of ischemic suffering of the flap, in particular type III and IV in patients who are smokers, diabetics or previously subjected to RT.

Nipple-sparing mastectomy

Nipple-sparing mastectomy (NSM) was born as a response to the difficulty of obtaining valid reconstruction of the nipple–areola complex (NAC) in terms of projection, position, form, size and color following modified radical or total mastectomy, or SSM. In a trial of 2002 Jabor et al. highlighted a low degree of satisfaction following NAC reconstruction; only 16% of the patients stated that they did not wish to resort to surgical revision of the NAC [12].

NSM was initially proposed as the treatment of choice for patients suffering from fibrocystic mastopathy, chronic mastitis, changes of breast parenchyma in trauma or multiple biopsies outcomes and family history for breast carcinoma. The quest for ever better esthetic outcomes, nurtured by patients' expectations, has led to investigating its safety so as to extend its indications [13].

The removal of the NAC during the course of a mastectomy is based on the presupposition that there may be hidden involvement of the NAC. This is involved in a percentage varying from 0 to 58% on the basis of size, position and multicentricity of the tumor, lymph node involvement and the presence of an extensive intraductal component. As in the case of SSM, also for NSM the literature that sought to evaluate its oncological safety was ample [13,14].

The studies conducted have made it clear that NAC conservation is a safe procedure when there is no clinical evidence of NAC or periareolar skin involvement, secretion or bleeding, when the tumor is of small dimensions, <2.5 cm, localized far from the areola, tumor–nipple distance >4 cm, and there is no lymph node involvement.

All these studies are based on histological analysis of the tissue removed following subcutaneous mastectomy or SSM without RT.

In the light of preliminary data on IORT following conservative surgery (ELIOT), Petit et al. [15] proposed NAC conservation in selected patients and candidates for mastectomy, subjected to IORT focussed on the NAC. Once the mastectomy has been completed a thin layer of retroareolar glandular tissue is removed and analyzed in the freezer; if this has a negative outcome, a dose of 16Gy is administered at NAC level. This has enabled NSM indications to be extended to patients with extensive and multicentric tumors or with widespread microcalcifications far from the NAC.

NSM is therefore proposed as a valid alternative to traditional mastectomy, offering in selected cases the same long-term survival and the possibility of immediate reconstruction with better esthetic outcomes. Moreover, this technique avoids patients having to undergo the multiple operations necessary to reconstruct the NAC, reducing costs in terms of the psychological and economic impact linked with reconstruction.

As for SSM, various types of incision have been proposed for NSM, too. The periareolar incision, laterally extended, permits easy access for dissection of the retroareolar ducts and lateral glandular tissue; the lateral extension of the incision aids dissection of the lateral margin of the large pectoral muscle, facilitating insertion of the cutaneous expansor; the transareolar incision, laterally extended, transareolar with medial and lateral extension, and at the level of the inframammary fold.

In 2007 Regolo et al. proposed new surgical access to reduce the risk of NAC necrosis and consequently of exposure of the expansor [16]. According to some studies the necrosis rate for the NAC varies from 2% to 20% depending on the technique and whether or not RT is applied. The vitality of the NAC is ensured by the vessels supplying the nipple, ducts and surrounding skin, but the NSM surgical technique envisages extensive retroareolar detachment necessary to obtain the most complete removal possible of breast tissue.

Periareolar incision very often damages vascularization, favoring cutaneous necrosis. The alternative proposed by Regolo provides for a vertical incision of 6–8 cm along the lateral profile of the breast. This permits easy access to the axillary lymph nodes, preserves NAC vascularization with vascular complications reduced to 2.8%, leaving a scar outcome not visible from the front. Lateral access also facilitates breast reconstruction with expansor/prosthesis.

The disadvantages connected with this new incision consist of difficult detachment of the medial quadrants and possible lateralization of the NAC due to scar retraction.

Skin Reducing Mastectomy

Skin reducing mastectomy may be defined as a variant of type IV SSM. This technique combines SSM with an immediate reduction in the cutaneous cover of the breast; it is based on the same oncological principles as SSM, but in addition a lower dermal flap is sculpted, and used to create a dermo-muscular pocket to ensure better covering of the expansor/prosthesis.

SSM has reduced the need of cutaneous expansion but in many cases the implant covering does not manage to be optimal especially at the level of the inframammary fold, where this may be found to lie immediately underneath the cutaneous cover [17].

In 1990 Bostwick proposed a change in SSM for the first time but did not meet with wide approval. In 2005 Nava et al. reported this technique with the name Skin Reducing Mastectomy, with the intention of reducing to a minimum the complications of SSM, the risk of prosthesic exposure due to ischemic suffering of the flap, and the loss of projection of the reconstructed breast in the lower quadrants.

The procedure is currently indicated for women with large or ptotic breasts who are candidates for skin sparing mastectomy for breast carcinoma or prophylaxis, obtaining excellent esthetic results, still more evident if combined with reductive mastoplasty or contralateral mastopexy [17].

The surgical technique combines the traditional incision for reductive mastoplasty, the Wise pattern, with the positioning of an inferior dermal flap. The pre-operative plan consists of tracing the new seat of the NAC along the hemi-clavicular line at a distance of 19–23 cm from the jugular vein. From this point two oblique lines of approximately 7 cm are traced forming an angle of 30°–90°, extended as far as the intersection with the inframammary fold.

The incision involves the whole thickness along the two oblique lines, but the epidermis only at the inframammary fold level. A small triangle of epidermis can be preserved at the level of the intersection point between the vertical and horizontal arms of the T to reduce cutaneous tension at the moment of suture. A dermal flap is positioned in the area between the fold and the two oblique lines and mastectomy performed preserving vascularization of the flap. When axillary lymphoadenectomy proves necessary, the same surgical access as the mastectomy can be used or a new incision made at the axillary level.

Once mastectomy has been concluded, an incision is made at the lateral margin of the large pectoral muscle and a deep sub-muscular pocket created under the large pectoral and serratus anterior muscles. The prosthesis is put into place and complete closure of the pocket is obtained thanks to three sutures: between the large pectoral muscles and the serratus anterior, between the large pectoral and the dermal flap and between the latter and the serratus anterior [17].

Conservative Surgery

In the last twenty years conservative therapy has become the chosen therapy for breast carcinoma in many cases. It includes:
- Quadrantectomy: removal of one quarter of the mammary gland, skin overlying the tumor, portion of areola and in depth the large pectoral muscle fascia. It may or may not be combined with axillary lymphoadenectomy
- Wide removal: removal of glandular tissue including the tumor and a margin of at least 1 cm of microscopically healthy parenchyma with or without overlying skin
- Tumorectomy: removal of the portion of mammary gland containing the tumor and the seat of previous biopsies. The overlying skin is usually conserved.

The treatment protocol is the subject of continuous study: the current trend is for patients with a favorable tumor/breast size relationship and with no risk factors for local recurrence (infiltration of margins, extended intraductal component) to be candidates for conservative surgery. It is usually followed by RT but in low-risk patients (post-menopause, tumors of small dimensions, peritumoral hematic or lymphatic, absence of extensive intraductal component) the indication is studied case by case. The introduction of neoadjuvant therapies able to reduce the dimensions of the tumor has enabled the indications to be widened also to tumors of large dimensions.

In the cases in which it has been applied, the technique has demonstrated the same rate of survival as mastectomy, though offering esthetic, functional and psychological advantages [18]. The problem conservative surgery has to face is to obtain the widest margins of excision possible and therefore reduce the risk of local recurrence but at the same time obtain a good esthetic result. When conservative therapy was introduced patients were satisfied that they could conserve their breast and above all the NAC. With the development and spread of conservative treatment a progressive increase in the esthetic expectations of patients has been witnessed. Ideally, conservative therapy should ensure a breast with a natural, "normal" appearance and no deformity or asymmetry.

Oncoplastic surgery, namely the application in conservative oncological surgery of techniques developed by plastic surgeons for plastic surgery of the breast, is able to offer a valid solution to the conflict between surgical radicality and cosmetic treatment.

Oncoplastic objectives are the local control of the tumor with an optimal esthetic and functional result. These are achieved by singling out the best surgical strategy and adapting it to the individual patient on the grounds of the seat and size of the tumor, tumor volume/breast volume relationship, shape and dimensions of the breast, and age and expectations of the patient [19]. For this reason pre-operative planning requires a multidisciplinary team: senologic surgeon, plastic surgeon, radiotherapist and radiologist, pathologist and physiotherapist.

Oncoplastic surgery is applied to breasts of medium-large dimensions, when more than 20% of the breast volume needs to be removed without having recourse to mastectomy. It is, however, contraindicated in patients with a T4 tumor, multicentric disease, widespread malignant microcalcifications and inflammatory carcinoma.

Plastic surgery offers a wide range of techniques for breast remodelling: the residual glandular defect can be remodelled thanks to local glandular flaps, superior or inferior pedicle mastoplasty, mastoplasty using the "L" technique, mastoplasty with the Benelli round block technique, with Grisotti advancement-rotation flaps, and with the possibility of NAC reimplantation.

This ideal result, however, is not achieved for all patients, and actually the initial indication for conservative surgery very often proves incorrect.

Clough et al. have proposed a classification of the esthetic sequelae of conservative surgery that can act as a guide for the evaluation and treatment of these patients [20].

- Type 1: General shape of breast conserved with no deformity but presence of asymmetry in shape and/or volume compared with the contralateral
- Type 2: Presence of deformity able to be corrected without recourse to mastectomy
- Type 3: Presence of severe deformity and possibility of recreating normal shape and contour.

For each type of defect the possible surgical treatment was proposed: Type 1, contralateral symmetrisation operations, repositioning of the NAC, scar revision, fold liposuction or lipofilling; Type 2 is the most difficult to correct and it is in these cases that foresight is needed requiring the collaboration of the plastic surgeon for the first operative session; Type 3, mastectomy and reconstruction with myocutaneous flaps.

In selected cases, so as to obtain an optimal esthetic result and reduce the number of operations, it is preferable to resort to SSM or NSM rather than conservative surgery, followed by immediate breast reconstruction and, if necessary, symmetrization of the contralateral breast.

Breast Reconstruction

The breast reconstruction operation has received a great stimulus in recent years due both to the substantial increase in demand but above all to the evidence that the reconstructive operation does not affect the course of the disease and does not interfere with subsequent therapies or diagnostic investigations. Its development has been favored not only by the evolution of mastectomy techniques, but by increasingly conservative therapeutic choices such as quandrantectomy, tumorectomy and wide resection. In its turn the development of reconstructive surgery has determined the progress of techniques already used, the introduction of new ones and not least the design of prosthetic implants with increasingly sophisticated shapes.

Breast reconstruction is currently considered a part of the integrated treatment for breast carcinoma. The main objectives of breast reconstruction are: creation of breast prominence with a volume as similar as possible to the contralateral one and conservation of symmetry, definition of the superior and inferior mammary pole, redefinition of the inframammary fold, and NAC reconstruction.

The techniques available today enable good results to be obtained in the majority of cases, also in poor local conditions. The choice of reconstructive technique constitutes the most important moment of breast reconstruction and results from a series of factors like the patient's age, expectations, the quality of tissue at the seat of the mastectomy, and shape and volume of the contralateral breast. Breast volume may be recreated with both allogenic and autologous material. The choice of technique depends predominantly on the conditions of the cutaneous and muscular tissue of the thoracic region. In 60–70% of cases reconstruction involves the insertion of a cutaneous expansor in a pocket positioned under the muscle. The progressive filling of the expansor with saline solution determines progressive distension of the integuments, thus favoring the creation of more natural breast prominence after replacement with the final prosthesis [21]. Reconstruction with allogenic material offers a series of advantages such as the possibility of using the skin of the breast region without having recourse to myocutaneous flaps at a distance, minimal scar outcomes, simplicity and speed of the surgical technique and reduced hospitalization period.

In 30% of cases, particularly following RT, reconstruction with autologous tissue is to be preferred [21]. The main myocutaneous flaps used in breast reconstruction are the transverse rectus abdominus myocutaneous (TRAM) flap introduced by Hartrampf in 1982 and used both as a pedicled flap or free (anastomosis between the inferior epigastric artery and the thoracodorsal artery, subscapular or internal breast), combined with or without prosthesis. The introduction of "perforator flaps", microsurgical flaps based on the perforating arteries, has enabled the TRAM to be positioned by skeletonizing the pedicle and perforating vessels, saving the rectus abdominis muscle (DIEP). In some cases reconstructions may involve the use of autologous tissue, such as the latissimus dorsi or the TRAM combined with the insertion of a prosthesis.

Breast symmetry is ensured by plastic surgery operations on the contralateral breast, additive/reductive mastoplasty, or mastopexy, which enable a check up of the breast tissue at the same time. The risk of contralateral tumor is in effect estimated by various studies as between 7 and 20% [22].

In the cases in which it has not been possible to safeguard the NAC, this is reconstructed at a later stage using local flaps for reconstruction of the nipple and tattooing to recreate the colour of the areola.

It should be emphasized that as far as choice of technique is concerned, in the event there is a choice between different options, it is always a good rule to adopt the less demanding technique for the patient, which will allow a rapid recovery limiting interference and delay of the therapies that might follow the operation. It is nowadays a consolidated opinion that when possible breast reconstruction should be immediate, namely it should begin at the same time as the demolitive operation. It is just as important that there be close collaboration between the oncological surgeon and the plastic surgeon within the sphere of a senology unit.

Radiotherapy and Timing of Breast Reconstruction

The choice of appropriate timing and reconstructive therapy proves fundamental for the purpose of maximizing the esthetic result and reducing the risk of complications to a minimum. The main determinant in the choice of timing of reconstruction is represented by RT.

Adjuvant RT is an integral part of conservative treatment for breast carcinoma at an initial stage and, following mastectomy, of post-operative treatment in advanced stages. RT is able to reduce the rate of locoregional recurrence by 20% on average following conservative surgery, and by 30% following mastectomy [23]. Even if the possibility of needing to perform RT may be stated before the operation, the need of RT cannot be decided until anatomopathological assessment of breast and lymph node tissue has been concluded. Neither the intraoperative examination of the sentinel lymph node by freezer nor the immunohistochemical techniques are able to single out all micrometastases. The rate of false negatives at the intraoperative examination is rather high, around 89%. Moreover, even if the sentinel lymph node proves positive and lymph node dissection is performed, the final number of lymph nodes involved and the extension of the tumor cannot be known until some days after the operation.

Some recent studies have picked out certain clinicopathological factors able to preoperatively single out among patients with clinically negative lymph nodes those with a greater risk of occult micrometastases. Patients aged 50 or less, patients with a tumor exceeding 2 cm in size, and patients with evidence of lymphovascular involvement at biopsy have pathological lymph node involvement in 67% of cases [24].

The indications for postoperative RT are: tumors of large dimensions or with cutaneous involvement (T3–T4) or with involvement of more than four lymph nodes. The state of the axillary lymph nodes is the real determinant whether postoperative RT is needed or not and consequently the choice of timing of reconstruction [24].

Problems connected with RT interference in the type of reconstruction performed are highly topical.

Immediate Reconstruction

The application of post-operative RT also in cases of initial stage of the tumor and the impossibility of selection of those patients requiring RT has made immediate reconstruction planning more difficult. In spite of the fact that it is the ideal choice for many patients, two problems exist for performing immediate reconstruction on patients who will then undergo RT. First, RT can invalidate the esthetic results of immediate reconstruction. Even though RT techniques have been perfected since the mid 1970s, they continue to cause problems in the healing of the surgical wound and capsular contracture phenomena.

Secondly, immediate breast reconstruction can create problems in the planning and design of irradiation fields. The slope of the breast profile, after reconstruction, hinders determination of the medial and lateral irradiation fields, with the risk of underdosage to certain regions of the thoracic wall. Moreover, the thickness of the thoracic wall is not uniform, causing a non-homogeneous distribution of the dose within the fields [24].

Clinical trials show that the effects of RT on the reconstructed breast are due to: dose administered, use of filters, dose distribution, use of tissue-equivalent materials (bolus) applied to the skin surface, and use of a radiation "boost" on the bed of the tumor.

Immediate breast reconstruction is now recognized as a safe procedure from the oncological point of view and is able to offer a series of advantages, such as better esthetic results compared with delayed reconstruction, attenuation of the sense of mutilation deriving from the mastectomy and a reduction in surgical times [22].

The procedure is usually proposed for patients with Stage 1 breast carcinoma, Stage 2 if they do not present an increased risk to the point of needing RT, and in patients undergoing prophylactic mastectomy.

Immediate reconstruction may make use both of myocutaneous flaps and allogenic material. When possible the surgeon's and patient's choice will fall on the use of the cutaneous expansor later substituted by the final prosthesis, or in those patients who refuse the second operation, on expanding prostheses. Usually after a mastectomy two-stage reconstruction is always recommended and only in some selected cases of small and non-ptotic breasts may the prosthesis be inserted from the start. The use of expansors is more and more common in immediate reconstructions and naturally requires a second intervention, but the final esthetic results are very good. It also enables a more precise choice of prosthesis size.

Achieving good esthetic results begins with the choice of type of patient adapting best to this type of operation. It is important to consider the patient's physiognomy, age, general conditions of health, diet, degree of sports activity carried out, tumor stage and therapies she will have to follow. Good results are obtained in bilateral reconstructions following prophylactic or subcutaneous mastectomies, in women with breasts of medium volume, not particularly ptotic. Contraindications in respect of the use of an expansor/prosthesis are the preoperative execution of RT, obesity, breasts of large dimensions or ptotic [25]. Subsequent assessment concerns the choice of cutaneous expander. A wide range of expansors are available on the market which differ in length, width and projection. The choice is usually guided by the features of the contralateral breast.

The cutaneous expander, after adequate preparation, is placed within the muscular pocket previously prepared and progressively brought to the desired volume. Positioning of the pocket may take place by the transpectoral or infrapectoral route; in the latter case the inferior fibers of the large pectoral muscle are disconnected. This type of approach permits greater definition of the inframammary fold favoring subsequent insertion of the prosthesis.

Planning of the second surgery session, approximately six months after the last expansion, begins with evaluation of the results obtained especially in terms of symmetry, volume and position of the inframammary fold. In this phase, as well as substituting the expansor with the final prosthesis, other procedures may be performed such as capsulotomy, to enlarge the capsule medially, laterally, below or, more rarely, above; capsulorapphia to reduce, on the other hand, the dimensions of the pocket. Still at the same operative session it is possible to perform remodelling of the contralateral breast depending on the patient's requests.

Deferred Reconstruction

This is usually performed from 3 to 6 months after mastectomy to permit complete healing of the surgical wound and completion of the adjuvant therapies. The state of the skin of the breast and the integrity of the large pectoral muscle are determinants in the choice between reconstruction with autologous or allogenic tissue. When possible immediate reconstruction is always to be preferred (Table 9.1).

Table 9.1 A comparison of the principal aspects of immediate and deferred breast reconstruction

Immediate reconstruction	Deferred reconstruction
Pocket completely submuscular with possibility of dividing inferior insertions of large pectoral	Subpectoral pocket becoming subcutaneous in inferolateral portions
One operative session subsequent to mastectomy	Two operative sessions necessary following mastectomy
Possible delay for adjuvant therapies	Oncological follow-up completed
Slow filling of expansor	Rapid filling of expansor
Possible after RT	Problematic after RT
Lower psychological impact	Higher psychological impact

RT, tumor plus radiotherapy

Past, Present and Future of Breast Prostheses

The real technological innovation of these recent years concerns the production of breast prostheses and expansors. The challenge in mammary reconstruction lies in the recreation of breast projection and the inframammary fold. Nowadays this can be done, and good symmetry can also be obtained thanks to the wide variety of prostheses on the market. Silicone breast prostheses have been used since 1963, but over time considerable development has been witnessed in the materials of the prosthetic envelope and its contents, in an attempt to improve tolerability and duration of their shape and profile. A table showing a summary of the main changes made in the production of breast prostheses has been proposed [26].

One of the recent innovations in the field of breast prostheses consists of the introduction of cohesive gel. The first prosthesis with cohesive gel was produced in 1993 and it continues to be the one most used in the world. Since then some changes

9

have been made to silicone gel, making it softer, but above all a number of shapes and profiles have become available, 12 different shapes for each volume. Prostheses are described for each volume with a letter (F: full, M: moderate, L: low) for their length and one for projection. In recent times extra projection has also been introduced indicated with the letter X. These prostheses are used in particular in breast reconstruction and for correcting congenital abnormalities or asymmetric breasts. The advantage of this type of prosthesis lies in the composition of the gel; this is able to maintain its own shape in the event a break occur in the envelope. Furthermore, inside the envelope a layer has been placed that is able to reduce spreading of the silicone to a minimum. The first data also show a decrease in the rate of capsular contracture. The reason is not yet known; some think this is due to less spreading of the silicone, others maintain it is due to the greater solidity of the prosthesis, able to inhibit contracture of the periprosthetic capsule. Certainly many other studies will be needed to find the answer to this query. The disadvantages connected with the use of these prostheses are prevalently the need for a surgical incision of at least 4.5–5.5 cm and the difficulty of insertion through a periareolar incision, given the non-deformability of the prosthesis, greater consistency and, not least, the certainly higher cost compared with the other silicone prostheses.

The continually increasing esthetic expectations and requests of patients have led to the development of a dual gel prosthesis. It is a prosthesis for reconstructive and additive mastoplasty unique of its kind, which responds perfectly to the doctor's requirements and the patient's desires. This is an innovative product characterized by the unique combination of two gels. The posterior part of the prosthesis is made of traditional cohesive gel, while the anterior part is made of a unique, highly cohesive gel. This feature ensures greater projection and support, highlighting the area of the NAC of the prosthesis. Apart from the unique combination of two gels, the posterior part of the prosthesis is concave to adapt better to the thoracic wall. It also has a tapering superior pole which, together with the concave base, reduces the space between the edge and the thoracic wall, minimizing palpability of the edges. Patients with a thin tissue cover above all gain advantage from this. As confirmation of the importance of the variety of choice, this prosthesis is available in 39 formats of different length, width and projection.

Expanding prostheses are also available on the market, consisting of an internal chamber with physiological solution and an external compartment containing silicone gel, which offer the possibility of modulating the final breast volume. In some cases they are used in reconstruction after SSM as they do not need expanding (Table 9.2).

Lipofilling

The idea of using adipose tissue as material for filling goes back to the end of the nineteenth century. It is currently applied in various spheres, in otolaryngology for laryngoplasty, in orthopedics as filling for bone defects, neurosurgery to obviate the loss of cerebrospinal fluids and again in general surgery to treat sphincter incontinence.

Table 9.2 Evolution of silicone breast prostheses

Implant generation	Production period	Characteristics
1st generation	1960s	Thick Shell (0.25mm average) thick, viscous gel, Dacron patch
2nd generation	1970s	Thin Shell (0.13mm average), less viscous gel, no patch
3rd generation	1960s–1992	Thick, silica reinforced, barrier coat shell
4th generation	1992–present	Stricter manufacturing standard, refined 3rd generation devices
5th generation	1993–present	Cohesive silicone gel filled devices

The first lipofilling application goes back to 1893, when Neuber used it to correct defects in the facial zone. In 1895 Czerny described a graft of adipose tissue, harvested from a dorsal lipoma, to fill minus outcome zone of benign breast tumor removal. In 1910 Lexer published his case studies on lipofilling with abdominal harvesting. In the first half of the fifties the spreading of studies showing poor vitality of reimplanted tissue at one year and the contemporary diffusion of prostheses halted its use, especially in the senologic sphere. With the introduction of liposuction, and Illouz' work published in 1983, adipose tissue harvesting became less invasive and greater quantities of lipoaspirate became available. Illouz' technique was subsequently modified by Fournier in 1985, who introduced the term liposculpture.

In 1995 Coleman worked out a rigid protocol for the phases of harvesting, purification and grafting of adipose tissue, demonstrating the long-term vitality of the transplant, particularly in facial rejuvenation surgery [27].

Over the years many authors have described lipofilling as a safe procedure, with low morbidity and ability to obtain good results in correcting defects in superficial tissues. Notwithstanding this, its spreading in the senologic sphere has been rather slow, due to the fact that each time procedures or technologies concerning the breast are spoken of, it needs to be considered whether they might interfere with the diagnosis of breast carcinoma or even be potentially able to cause it.

Currently lipofilling is considered in the same way as the other techniques for reconstructive breast surgery; the studies underway on post-mastectomy breast reconstruction with an adipose transplant only demonstrate this.

It can be used after demolitive surgery to correct defects in volume, shape and projection in breasts reconstructed both with alloplastic and autologous material; in the literature there have been reports of encouraging results in treating grade 3 and 4 recurring capsular contracture according to Becker, combined with capsulotomy. It also constitutes a valid solution for minimal/moderate defects in conservative surgery outcomes [27]. The most innovative concept concerning lipofilling is that introduced by Rigotti according to which the transfer of adipose tissue should not be considered mere filling but a supply of adipose stem cells to the receiving tissues, with the result of obtaining neovascularisation and an improvement in trophism of the tissues treated. The results of Rigotti's studies on radiodermal lesion treatment have been widely borrowed by the senologic sphere for the treatment of cutaneous radiodystrophy in radiation therapy outcomes [28].

Lipofilling may be carried out under local anesthetic with light sedation and may be combined with other breast reconstruction operations, such as NAC reconstruction, symmetrization of the contralateral breast, and liposuction of the inframammary fold.

Subcutaneous adipose tissue is usually harvested by liposuction with a syringe or aspirator from the abdomen and hips, as these regions have a higher content of progenitor and stem cells. The processing of lipoaspirate, necessary to remove the products of cell rupture and other contaminants like blood, local anesthetics and adrenalin, may be performed by manual lavage with physiological solution or by centrifugation at 50 g per 2 min. Positioning takes place using blunt cannulas with a diameter of between 14 and 17 gauge connected to syringes of 1–5 or 10 mL. The adipose tissue is injected in small quantities on different planes and trajectories while the cannula is being withdrawn [29].

The main contraindication of lipofilling consists obviously of the absence of an adipose panicle at the abdominal, gluteal or trochanteric level and consequent impossibility of harvesting, bearing in mind moreover the double 30% rule: 30% of the volume harvested is lost during processing and 30% of the volume injected is reabsorbed at a distance of approximately 4 months.

References

1. Fisher B, Jeong JH, Anderson S et al (2002) Twenty-five-year follow-up of a randomized trial comparing radical mastectomy, total mastectomy, and total mastectomy followed by irradiation. N Eng J Med 347: 567–575
2. Manasseh DME, Willey SC (2006) Invasive carcinoma: mastectomy and staging the axilla. In: Spear SL (ed) Surgery of the breast. Vol. 1. 2nd edn. Lippincott Williams & Wilkins, Philadelphia, pp 132–139
3. Early Breast Cancer Trialists Collaborative Group (EBCTCG) (2005) Effect of radiotherapy and of differences in the extent of surgery for early breast cancer on local recurrence and 15 years survival: an overview of randomised trials. Lancet 366:2087–2106
4. Schwartz GF, Giuliano AE, Veronesi U (2002) The Consensus Conference Committee. In: Proceeding of the consensus conference on the role of sentinel node biopsy in carcinoma of the breast. April 19-22, 2001, Philadelphia. Cancer 94:2542–2551
5. Tafra L, Lannin DR, Swanson MS et al (2001) Multicenter trial of sentinel node biopsy for breast cancer using both technetium sulphur colloid and isosulfan blue dye. Ann Surg 233:51–59
6. Sandrucci S, Casalegno PS, Percivale P et al (1999) Sentinel lymph node mapping and biopsy for breast cancer: a review of the literature relative to 479 procedures. Tumori 85:425–434
7. Simmons RM, Fish SK, Gayle L et al (1999) Local and distant recurrence rates in skin-sparing mastectomies compared with non-skin-sparing mastectomies. Ann Surg Oncol 6: 676–681
8. Kroll SS, Khoo A, Singletary E et al (1999) Local recurrence risk after skin-sparing and conventional mastectomy: a 6-year follow-up. Plast Reconstr Surg 104:421–425

9. Toth BA, Forley BG, Calabria R (1999) Retrospective study of the skin-sparing mastectomy in breast reconstruction. Plast Reconstr Surg 104:77–84
10. Datta G, Carlucci S, Bussone R (2008) Star and comet incisions for skin sparing mastectomy. J Plast Reconstr Aesth Surg [Epub ahead of print]
11. Skoll PJ, Hudson DA (2002) Skin sparing mastectomy using a modified Wise pattern. Plast Reconstr Surg 110:214–217
12. Jabor MA, Shayani P, Collins DR Jr et al (2002) Nipple–areola reconstruction: satisfaction and clinical determinants. Plast Reconstr Surg 110:457–463
13. Chung AP, Sacchini V (2008) Nipple sparing mastectomy: where are we now? Surg Oncol 17:261–266
14. Simmons RM, Brennan M, Christos P et al (2002) Analysis of nipple areolar involvement with mastectomy: can the areola be preserved? Ann Surg Oncol 9:165–168
15. Petit JY, Veronesi U, Orecchia R et al (2006) Nipple-sparing mastectomy in association with intraoperative radiotherapy (ELIOT) a new type of mastectomy for breast cancer. Breast Cancer Res Treat 96:47–51
16. Regolo L, Ballardini B, Gallarotti E et al (2008) Nipple sparing mastectomy: an innovative skin incision for an alternative approach. Breast 17:8–11
17. Querci della Rovere G, Nava M, Bonomi R et al (2008) Skin reducing mastectomy with breast reconstruction and sub-pectoral implants. Plast Reconstr Surg 61:1303–1308
18. Grisotti A, Calabrese C (2006) Conservative treatment of breast cancer: reconstructive problems. In: Spear SL (ed) Surgery of the breast. Vol. 1. 2nd edn. Lippincott Williams & Wilkins, Philadelphia, pp 147–216
19. Clough KB, Lewis JS, Couturaud B et al (2003) Oncoplastic techniques allow extensive resections for breast conserving therapy of breast carcinomas. Ann Surg 237:26–34
20. Clough KB, Thomas SS, Couturaud B et al (2004) Reconstruction after conservative treatment for breast cancer: cosmetic sequelae classification revisited. Plast Reconstr Surg 114:1743–1753
21. Spear SL, Boehmler JH, Bogue DP, Mafi AA (2008) Options in reconstructing the irradiated breast. Plast Reconstr Surg 122:379–388
22. Petit JY, Rietjens M, Garusi C (2001) Breast reconstructive techniques in cancer patients: which ones, when to apply, which immediate and long term risks? Oncol Hematol 38:231–239
23. Richetti A (2008) Conventional, intraoperative, partial radiotherapy and aesthetic outcomes. In: Proceeding of conference on oncoplastic surgery of the breast cancer. Rapallo 20–21 Oct
24. Kronovitz SJ, Robb GL (2006) Controversies regarding immediate reconstruction: aesthetic risks of radiation. In: Spear SL (ed) Surgery of the breast. Vol. 1. 2nd edn. Lippincott Williams & Wilkins, Philadelphia, pp 679–699
25. Spear SL, Schwarz K (2006) Prosthetic reconstruction in radiated breast. In: Spear SL (ed) Surgery of the breast Vol. 1. 2nd edn. Lippincott Williams & Wilkins, Philadelphia, pp 515–530
26. Adams WP Jr, Potter JK (2006) Breast implant: materials and manufacturing past, present and future. In: Spear SL (ed) Surgery of the breast. Vol. 1. 2nd edn. Lippincott Williams & Wilkins, Philadelphia, pp 424–437
27. Missana MC, Laurent I, Barreau L, Balleyguier C (2007) Autologous fat transfer in reconstructive breast surgery: indications, technique and results. J Can Surg 33:685–690
28. Rigotti G, Marchi A, Galie M et al (2007) Clinical treatment of radiotherapy tissue damage by lipoaspirate transplant: a healing process mediated by adipose-derived adult stem cells. Plast Reconstr Surg 119:1409–1422
29. Chan CW, McCulley SJ, Macmillan RD (2008) Autologous fat transfer – a review of the literature with a focus on breast cancer surgery. J Plast Reconstr Aesthet Surg 61:1438–1448

Transplants in Surgical Oncology

10

M. Salizzoni, G. Carbonaro, L. Repetto

Introduction

In 1967 Thomas Starzl performed the first orthotopic liver transplant (OLT) in Denver. Since 1990 OLT has been the main therapy for every form of terminal liver failure, including hepatocellular carcinoma (HCC). In 1996 Mazzaferro published the results obtained on selected patients affected with HCC. He showed a 4 year survival rate of 75%, comparable to the rate obtained on patients who were transplanted for non tumoral pathology (78.3%) [1].

These results have encouraged the use of OLT for other neoplasms. Today, transplant is considered a possible treatment for hepatoblastoma (HB), hepatic epithelioid hemangioendothelioma (HEHE) and for the neuroendocrine tumor metastasis. Cholangiocarcinoma (hilar and peripheral) and adenocarcinoma metastasis of the colon currently represent a contraindication.

Unlike HCC which originates on a cirrhotic liver, other cancers arise in healthy livers; therefore, the indication for transplant is exclusively placed for neoplastic pathology and it is not placed for the underlying hepatopathy. For this reason it is fundamental to find a graft with a precise timing from an oncological point of view, for example, by taking advantage of the post-chemotherapy temporal window.

Two main issues of transplant have to be highlighted. On the one hand there is the lack of organs and on the other there is immunosuppression which helps both the onset of relapses and possible de novo tumors. Although much progress has been made in terms of immune therapy, the insertion of a patient affected with tumor in the waiting list cannot disregard the data obtained in the literature. The new mTOR pharmaceutical inhibitors and Sorafenib could play a fundamental role, but further research is necessary to expand transplant indications for oncological pathology.

M. Salizzoni (✉)
Liver Translantation Unit – General Surgery 8, S. Giovanni Battista University Hospital, Turin, Italy

New Technologies in Surgical Oncology. Antonio Mussa (Ed.)
© Springer-Verlag Italia 2010

Hepatocellular Carcinoma (HCC) on Cirrhosis

From an oncological point of view, HCC certainly represents the most frequent indication for liver transplant. With about 700,000 new cases every year around the world, it represents the fifth cause of death in the world from cancer as well as the first cause of death in the world among cirrhotic patients. In fact 90% of these cancers originate from cirrhotic livers. Each one of these diseases (HCC and cirrhosis) has its own morbidity and mortality rate.

The prognosis of HCC differs depending on the stage in which the HCC is diagnosed. For each stage there is a different treatment. Various therapeutic systems have been proposed in the literature. Currently, the most used therapeutic system is the one proposed by the BCLC group.

Although the discussion on the best treatment for patients in the "very early" stage is still ongoing, it is accepted that OLT is the gold standard for patients who are included in the Milan criteria (one nodule <5 cm or up to 3 nodes with the major node having a maximum diameter of 3 cm). In fact, the survival rate results and the 5 year disease free survival rate results of 70% and 83%, respectively, have made these criteria universal. To achieve these results, patients in the early stage are subject to transplant even if they are Child A. In February 2002, the MELD (model for end-stage liver disease) score was created to identify priority criteria for access to transplant for patients in the waiting list. This score is exclusively based on hepatic function data, thus the issue of the drop-out of patients affected with HCC but with good residual hepatic function has been placed. This issue has been resolved by allocating a supplementary score to HCC patients. The good results on patients who have been transplanted while in the early stage have encouraged the expansion of the Milan criteria as well as the criteria proposed by the University of California, San Francisco (UCSF) [2]. However, this attempt to expand the Milan criteria raises the main issue of the organ shortage, with the consequence of an increase in both waiting time and drop-out of patients in the waiting list.

Living donor liver transplantation (LDLT) has been proposed to expand the availability of the organs. Currently the indications on LDLT are the same as those on the cadaveric donor. In fact it is not yet clear whether the results obtained with this method are better than those obtained with livers from cadaveric donors. Moreover, the mortality problem reported in the literature of 0.5% on the recipient and the 15% morbidity rate is still a major problem. The use of marginal livers is certainly the way to expand the pool of organs mostly used in Italy. In this country patients in the early stage are transplanted even though the research to validate the expansion of the Milan criteria has been undertaken. Patients outside of the Milan criteria are only transplanted within a controlled trial. The use of Sorafenib (multikinase inhibitor), has shown survival benefits in patients with advanced HCC [3]. Perhaps it can play a role similar to a neoadjuvant therapy, but more studies need to be carried out.

Fibrolamellar Hepatocellular Carcinoma (FLHCC)

Fibrolamellar hepatocellular carcinoma (FLHCC) is an uncommon tumor that differs from hepatocellular carcinoma (HCC) in demographics, condition of the affected liver, tumor markers and prognosis. The clinical presentation of patients with FLHCC is variable. Use of percutaneous biopsy (FNAB) is beneficial if there is diagnostic uncertainty about the radiologic diagnosis (US, CT, MRI). Tumor resectability is the basis of curative therapy for patients with FLHCC; adequate tumor clearance may be accomplished by major resection, without the fear of post-surgical liver failure; however, at the most these tumors are resectable in only one-third of newly diagnosed patients. OLT has been used in patients with unresectable FLHCC [4–6]. Currently OLT is indicated when the tumor is limited to the liver without lymph node involvement.

Hepatoblastoma (HB)

This is the most frequent liver tumor in pediatric age with an incidence peak in the first 3 years of life. HB is most likely to originate from the liver's pluripotent cells during embryonic life. There are different histotypes, each with its own prognosis as highlighted from the SIOP (International Society of Paediatric Oncology). The fetal morphological type has the best prognosis. The modality of the clinical presentation is variable, generally it presents as an abdominal mass and there rarely is an alteration of the laboratory investigations of hepatic functionality.

Rupture may occur, which manifests in hemoperitoneum. In terms of laboratory work-up, 70% of cases reveal high levels of alpha-fetoprotein. This marker allows the identification of early relapses as well as evaluating the response to neoadjuvant treatments. A value of alpha-fetoprotein <100 is considered a negative prognostic factor. In children younger than 6 months old the alpha-fetoprotein and the alpha-fetoprotein fetal residual toned to be distinguished. The possible differential diagnosis with other tumors such as HCC, HEHE or angiosarcoma and the different prognostic results based on the histological type justify the performance of a diagnostic biopsy before any treatment. Such a biopsy should be performed through healthy parenchyma, with the objective of preventing tumor seeding. Even for this pathology there are different staging systems. In Europe, the most used system is the one proposed by SIOP called PRETEXT. This evaluates the extension of the tumor before any treatment takes place, based on what the imaging exams highlight. The number of hepatic segments touched by the tumor are evaluated, as well as any vascular infiltration, lymph node metastasis and/or extrahepatic metastases. Based on the histological type, on the alpha-fetoprotein value and on the PRETEXT stage, patients are stratified into high risk (HR) and standard risk (SR). HR patients have alpha-fetoprotein values <100, unfavorable histological type such as undifferentiated subtype, PRETEXT IV (involvement of all the hepatic segments) or patients presenting vascular infiltrations and/or lymph node metastasis or in any other organ. The surgery resection R0 is the chosen treatment since it can guarantee a 10-year survival rate of 80% [7]. Immediately after diagnosis, about 60% of the patients are not ready to be resected, but fortunately this tumor is particularly sensitive to chemotherapy with cisplatin. This drug is used as a neoadjuvant with the objective of reducing the tumoral mass and allowing R0 surgery resection. Candidates for the resection are PRETEXT I and II patients as long as a resection margin of at least 1 cm can be guaranteed. All other patients are subject to chemotherapeutic neoadjuvant treatment. All remaining PRETEXT IV patients or PRETEXT III patients non-resectable after CT are subject to transplantation. The presence of extrahepatic metastasis is not a contraindication to the transplantation as long as they are resectable with R0 margin. OLT timing is fundamental, as it has to be performed within a few weeks from the last chemotherapy cycle. This requires a rapid access to the organ, and if this is not possible, LDLT has to be considered. OLT is a possible treatment also for patients who have been incompletely resected and present a disease relapse even if results in these patients are not good (30% at 6 years of age, rescue OLT) and for patients presenting hepatic insufficiency after chemotherapy and/or surgery resection [8].

Hepatic Epithelioid Hemangioendothelioma (HEHE)

This is a rare tumor which mainly affects young women. It originates from epithelial cells of the blood vessels and its main characteristic is slow growth, while bilobar involvement often does not allow resection. Liver transplantation on these patients has shown satisfactory results with a 5-year survival rate of 55%. The presence of extrahepatic metastasis is not a contraindication to transplantation.

Angiosarcoma

This is a very aggressive tumor which mainly affects the male sex, and has an average survival of 6 months. Considering the hypervascular nature of this tumor, generally the mode of presentation is by bleeding. This happens either because the tumor ruptures or because of thrombocytopenia which is secondary to a coagulopathy caused by the tumor itself. In contrast to HEHE this tumor represents an absolute contraindication to transplantation due to the low results linked to such aggressive neoplastic behavior.

Cholangiocarcinoma (CC)

Cholangiocarcinoma is a relatively rare tumor. In fact it accounts for 3% of gastrointestinal tract neoplasms and 10% of hepatic neoplasms. CCs arise from bile duct epithelium and are generally divided into peripheral type (from intrahepatic bile ducts) and extrahepatic (from extrahepatic bile ducts, including Klatskin tumor). In the therapy of hilar cholangiocarcinoma, the most favorable survival rates over the long-term are achieved by a surgical concept involving a no-touch-technique, en-bloc-resection and tumor-free margins. The 5-year survival rate in these patients is 61% [9]. Thanks to the transplant potential which guarantees R0 margins, it has also been proposed as a treatment for cholangiocarcinoma. The results have not been encouraging, showing 5-year survival rates of 25%. However, the best results have been obtained on patients with stage I tumors, i.e., on patients in whom surgery resection is still possible. At present, peripheral and extrahepatic CCs represent a contraindication to liver transplantation. However, a study done by the Mayo Clinic group has highlighted a disease free survival with a median follow-up of 37 months of 92% for patients accurately selected, treated with radiotherapy and neoadjuvant chemotherapy and liver transplantation [10]. A substantial drop-out rate from this neoadjuvant regimen due to tumor progression or treatment related complications is still a problem. Currently patients with CCs should be transplanted only in the setting of a controlled trial.

Liver Metastases from Neuroendocrine Tumors

Neuroendocrine tumors (NET) commonly metastasize to the liver. Neuroendocrine liver metastases (LM) frequently have an indolent clinical course in comparison with other gastrointestinal metastases. The metastases can be limited to the liver for prolonged periods of time. Many patients are asymptomatic, others have hormonal syndromes that can be controlled with long-acting somatostatin analogs. When there is bilobar disease, survival is limited with 5-year survival of only 30%. Although many treatments have been proposed, the optimal management is still ill defined. The spectrum of liver surgery comprises complete resection, palliative cytoreductive resection and liver transplantation. When possible R0 resection is the treatment of choice, eventually using portal embolization to induce hypertrophy of the remaining left liver before right hepatectomy. Although there is no evidence for the usefulness of liver transplantation in the treatment of metastases from NET, there are several single-centre studies that show an improved 5-year survival rate. OLT is reserved for selected patients with aggressive and not resectable tumors without extrahepatic disease. Reliable liver transplantation selection criteria remain unknown. Current data suggest that under 50 years age, prior resection of the primary tumor and primary tumor with low Ki67 proliferation index are favorable prognostic factors for the outcome of liver transplantation [11,12]. It has also been suggested that carcinoid from the small intestine may have a better outcome than NET arising from the pancreas [13]. With a good selection, it is possible to have an overall 5-year survival of 80% [14]. Many more data are needed to validate this indication, and currently there are no guidelines.

Liver Metastases from Colorectal Cancer

Liver transplantation for non resectable liver metastases from colorectal cancer was abandoned in 1994 on account of high recurrence rates. However, in 2005, successful long-term survival following LT for metastatic gastrointestinal tumors in two patients was reported (patients were alive with no tumor evidence at 18 and 69 months respectively [14]). At present this remains a contraindication to liver transplantation.

The Role of mTOR

The incidence of de novo post transplant malignancies have been reduced by the use of drugs named mammalian target of rapamycin inhibitor (mTOR). Several studies have shown that mTOR are effective and well tolerated in orthotopic liver transplant patients with hepatocellular carcinoma (HCC), achieving excellent survival and disease-free intervals, particularly with extended criteria tumors. Regression of metastatic HCC and other tumors and various forms of post transplant lymphoproliferative diseases have occurred after mTOR conversion. Unfortunately, there is not a single report on the prospective clinical trial designed for looking at the effect of mTOR in transplant recipients [15]. Further studies are needed to validate the use of this drug as a cornerstone for immunosuppressive therapy for transplant patients.

Kidney Transplant and Oncology

(Guidelines of The European Association of Urology Regarding Kidney Transplant (Updated in March 2004) "Donor Selection and Exclusion Criteria": Malignant Tumor).

Active neoplasms, history of breast carcinoma, melanoma, leukemia or lymphoma in donors are absolute contraindications for the transplant. If a potential donor has undergone a brain hemorrhage of unknown origin, the presence of metastases must be excluded as the cause of intracranial bleeding.

With other types of neoplasm, if less than 10 years has elapsed since the treatment, only "life-saving" transplants are recommended. Kidney transplants have been successfully carried out with small, low grade and fully removed carcinomas. These recipients need to be strictly monitored during follow-up.

Special Exceptions for Malignant Neoplasm

Donation is not contraindicated for the following tumors:
- Basal cell carcinoma
- Non-metastatic spinocellular skin carcinoma

- Cervical carcinoma *in situ*
- Vocal cord carcinoma *in situ*

There is no agreement for the use of donors with stage Ta G1 (TNM) bladder TCC. Prostate cancer screening is different in every country and is usually advised only when there are valid reasons.

Donors that have the following low-grade brain tumors (1 and 2), can be considered as kidney donors:

- Low-grade astrocytoma
- Pituitary adenoma
- Epidermoid cysts
- Colloid cysts of the third ventricle
- Pilocytic astrocytomas and ependymomas
- Low-grade oligodendrogliomas
- Gangliomas, gangliocytomas
- Benign meningiomas
- Craniopharyngiomas
- Hemangioblastomas (non associated with Von Hippel Lindau disease)
- Acoustic nerve schwannoma
- Pineocytomas
- Well-differentiated teratomas

Potential recipients with the following high-grade tumors (grade 3 and 4) can undergo a transplant only in the event of clinical urgency:

- Anaplastic astrocytoma
- Anaplastic oligodendroglioma (Schmidt C and D)
- Malignant ependymoma
- Gliomatosis cerebri
- Glioblastoma multiforme
- Pineoblastoma
- Medulloblastoma
- Germ cell tumor (except well-differentiated teratomas)
- Anaplastic and malignant meningiomas
- Intracranial sarcomas
- Chordomas
- Primary cerebral lymphomas.

Patients suffering from cerebral neoplasms of any grade who have undergone a VP shunt must be excluded due to the high risk of severe dissemination of neoplastic cells through the shunt.

Complication of Immunodepression after Transplant

The incidence of neoplasm in transplanted patients is higher than in the general population. It is an important cause of morbidity and mortality in transplanted patients. The presence of a neoplasm can be due to:

- A previous neoplasm in the recipient, whether known or latent
- Transmission of a neoplasm from the donor to the recipient
- Growth of a new tumor in the recipient.

Previous Neoplasm in the Recipient, Whether Known or Latent

Active neoplasms in the recipient are a contraindication for transplant due to the risk of metastases and dissemination, while a personal history of a previous neoplasm does not always exclude the possibility of a transplant. Nevertheless, when the disease is not active it may be difficult to assess when the patient can be a candidate for the transplant.

The risk of recurrence depends on the type of tumor and the time that has elapsed between the cancer treatment and the transplant. If the waiting time is shorter than 2 years the risk of recurrence is 53%. However, if more than 5 years have elapsed since therapy, the risk drops to 13%, while between 2 and 5 years the risk is 34%.

For many tumors the waiting period should be 2 years, but there are numerous exceptions.

Less than two years:
- Skin basal cell carcinoma
- Totally removed squamous cell carcinoma
- Incidentally diagnosed renal cell carcinoma (RCC)
- In situ or low grade bladder carcinoma
- Small and single focal neoplasm

More than two years:
- Large or symptomatic RCC
- Invasive bladder carcinoma
- Prostate carcinoma
- Breast carcinoma
- Malignant melanoma
- Colorectal carcinoma
- Uterine cervix invasive carcinoma.

Relapses in the first two years have been observed in Wilms' tumor, symptomatic RRC, bladder carcinoma and non-melanoma skin tumor. Although a 5-year period can eliminate most relapses, this is not an absolute rule, especially in the elderly. A 2-year wait would eliminate 91% of relapses of Wilms' tumor, 64% of bladder neoplasms and 61% of symptomatic RCC relapses. However, this 2-year period would eliminate 13% of relapses of colorectal carcinoma and 40% of prostate carcinoma.

The risk of relapses of previous carcinomas after kidney transplant is:
- Low risk (0–10%) – incidental RCC, lymphoma, testicle, uterine, cervical and thyroid carcinomas
- Medium risk (10–25%) – endometrial carcinoma, Wilms' tumor, colon, breast and prostate carcinomas
- High risk (>25%) – bladder carcinoma, sarcomas, skin carcinoma, symptomatic RCC, myelomas.

Immunosuppression can stimulate the growth of dormant metastases and the patient can develop relapses of neoplasms treated 5 years before the transplant. While many centers require a disease-free period of more than two years before the transplant for the majority of the tumors, the waiting period should be distinct for every tumor. A shorter waiting period could be sufficient in many tumors, recommending a disease-free period of more than one year. However with invasive neoplasms with an unfavorable prognosis, a 5-year period might be necessary.

Those patients who are on a waiting list for a transplant for a long time should be evaluated on a yearly basis to rule out the development of new neoplasms which might preclude or delay the transplant.

PSA-positive Donor

The determination of total PSA and the ratio of free PSA/total PSA is recommended in males over the age of 50. The examination should be carried out on a sample of serum taken when the patient is first hospitalized, or possibly before the bladder catheter is applied in the critical area. For patients over the age of 50, without a positive medical history for prostate neoplastic pathology, the following behavior is implemented:

- Total PSA values lower than 4 ng/mL allow organ removal for the purpose of transplant
- Total PSA values lower than 10 ng/mL associated with a value of the free PSA/total PSA ratio higher than 25% allow organ removal for the purpose of transplant.

Higher values must be evaluated in a broader context, considering that the PSA value can be altered by factors that are not related to the presence of a neoplasm, and that a PSA value higher than 10 ng/mL represents an indicative value. If pathological values are found, a urology test will be required with a transrectal ultrasound scan if possible, accompanied by a biopsy if nodules with suspicion of neoplasm are found.

Should the case be difficult to interpret, it is advisable to contact the experts of the National Transplant Centre (second opinion).

In the event of an adenocarcinoma confined within the prostate gland and extending to one or both lobes, if the Gleason score does not reveal any sample with predominant grade 4, the donor is considered at standard risk. Informed consent is necessary when one or more samples show a Gleason score with predominant grade 4 and/or show 10 clinical, instrumental or histopathological signs of local extension of the neoplasm outside the prostate gland. In this case "increased but acceptable risk" procedures are applied.

The "acceptable risk" group includes only cases with ascertained lymph node or distant metastases.

When a histopathological check-up is not possible, the PSA density method can be used. The density is determined by dividing the serum PSA values by the weight of the prostate. The weight of the prostate can be established using the volumetric measurements obtained with the transrectal ultrasound scan with the following formula:

length width height (π/6)

If the PSA *density* is ≤0.01 ng/mL/g the donor is considered at standard risk. In the event of higher values, if there is no support for the definition and stratification of the specific risk profile of metastases spread (frozen section examination of the prostate gland or sextant needle biopsy of the prostate fragments) if pathological PSA values are found, the National Transplant Centre can authorize the use of organs for urgent recipients following informed consent, keeping in mind the type of organs donated as well as the clinical features of the recipient.

References

1. Mazzaferro V, Regalia E, Doci R et al (1996) Liver transplantation for the treatment of small hepatocellular carcinomas in patients with cirrosi. N Engl J Med 334:693
2. Yao FY, Ferrel L, Bass NM et al (2001) Liver transplantation for hepatocellular carcinoma: expansion of tumor size limits does not adversely impact survival. Hepatology 33:1394
3. Llovet JM, Bruix J (2008) Molecular targeted therapies in hepatocellular carcinoma. Hepatology 48:1312–1327
4. Ringe B, Wittekind C, Weimann A et al (1992) Results of hepatic resection and transplantation for fibrolamellar carcinoma. Surg Gynecol Obstet 175:299–305
5. El Gazzaz G, Wong W, El Hadary MK et al (2000) Outcome of liver resection and transplantation for fibrolamellar hepatocellular carcinoma. Transpl Int 13[Suppl 1]:S406-S409
6. Schlitt HJ, Neipp M, Weimann A et al (1999) Recurrence patterns of hepatocellular and fibrolamellar carcinoma after liver transplantation. J Clin Oncol 17:324–331
7. Otte JB, de Ville de Goyet J (2005) The contribution of transplantation to the treatment of liver tumors in children. Semin Pediat Surg 14:233–238
8. Otte JB, Prichard J, Arason DC et al (2004) Liver transplantation for hepatoblastoma: results from the International Society of Pediatric Oncology (SIOP) study SIOPEL 1 and review of the world experience. Pediatr Blood Cancer 452:74–83
9. Jonas S, Benckert C, Thelen A et al (2008) Radical surgery for hilar cholangiocarcinoma. Eur J Surg Oncol 34:263–271
10. De Vreede I, Steers JL, Burch PA et al (2000) Prolonged disease-free survival after orthotopic liver transplantation plus adjuvant chemoirradiation for cholangiocarcinoma. Liver Transpl 6:309–316
11. Rosenau J, Bahr MJ, von Wasielewski R et al (2002) Ki67, E-cadherin, and p53 as prognostic indicators of long-term outcome after liver transplantation for metastatic neuroendocrine tumors. Transplantation 73:386–394
12. Coppa J, Pulvirenti A, Schiavo M et al (2001) Resection versus transplantation for liver metastases from neuroendocrine tumors. Transplant Proc 33:1537–1539
13. Cahlin C, Friman S, Ahlman H et al (2003) Liver transplantation for metastatic neuroendocrine tumor disease. Transpl Proc 35:809–810
14. Cameron S, Ramadori G, Fuzesi L et al (2005) Successful liver transplantation in two cases of metastatic gastrointestinal stromal tumor. Transplantation 2005:80 283–284
15. Monaco AP (2009) The role of mTOR inhibitors in the management of posttransplant malignancy. Transplantation 87:157–163

Locoregional Therapies and Surgical Oncology

11

C. R. Rossi, A. Comandone, A. Veltri

Introduction

The natural history of solid neoplasms starts as a confined disease in a specific anatomical area. This period varies greatly in length and involves carcinoma in situ as well as the stage I–II of the disease. In localized disease surgery is the mainstay. Radiotherapy can play a curative role in specific situations, but in general, together with chemotherapy it is an adjuvant treatment.

After metastatic spread the roles are generally reversed and chemotherapy as systemic therapy becomes the most important either in a curative or palliative setting. Sometimes, even in stage IV the tumor can be confined to a single organ such as the liver in colorectal cancer, the peritoneum in ovarian carcinoma, or the lung in bone and soft tissue sarcomas. This situation is called oligometastatic state and locoregional therapy has a good chance of being effective.

In contrast, in many other solid tumors metastatic involvement is a clear expression of a generalized evolution, such as liver metastases in breast cancer, peritoneal seeding in pancreatic carcinoma or contralateral involvement in lung cancer. In these latter cases the exclusive treatment of the metastases would have little benefit for the patient. In these situations systemic chemotherapy is the only useful therapy, at least with a palliative aim.

Nonetheless, the fact that in a minority of cancers locoregional therapies can be useful even in locally advanced or metastatic disease opens up an important possibility of treatment in specific settings.

Under the definition of locoregional therapies we include different approaches:
1. Techniques developed to increase the drug concentration in a specific area of the body through the blood supply: intra-arterial therapies, isolated limb perfusion, portal therapy [1,2]

C.R. Rossi (✉)
Sarcoma and Melanoma Unit, Clinica Chirurgica II, University of Padua, Padua, Italy

New Technologies in Surgical Oncology. Antonio Mussa (Ed.)
© Springer-Verlag Italia 2010

2. Techniques determining ischemia of the tumor blood supply: transarterial chemoembolisation (TACE), hepatic artery ligature
3. Techniques which directly expose the tumor cells localized into a natural cavity to a higher concentration of cytotoxic drug: intraperitoneal, intrapleural, intraventricular and intrathecal therapies [3]
4. Techniques that determine the immediate destruction of tumor nodules using physical or chemical approaches instead of drug action: alcoholization, radiofrequency, cryotherapy, radioisotopes, brachytherapy [4].

All the abovementioned therapies have two specific goals: increase the cell-kill activity on the tumor and decrease the toxicities on normal tissues.

The debated and critical points of locoregional treatments, after more than 40 years of worldwide experience are:

1. Limited diffusion and homogeneity of the techniques due to the complexity of the appliances, the long training required by the clinician to acquire the necessary expertise, and the elevated costs of many of the aforementioned techniques
2. Few randomized studies comparing locoregional and systemic therapies in common settings
3. The recent introduction in clinical oncology of so-called targeted therapies aimed at specific molecules or pathways in cancer cells in order to overcome the problem of drug concentration.

In conclusion, locoregional therapies play a valuable role in the global treatment of cancer. They should not be seen in antagonism with systemic therapy which still covers the large majority of cancer care, but rather as an important synergistic action in a modern, multidisciplinary approach.

Patient selection, the accurate definition of the role of systemic and local therapy, and the best synchronization of the two approaches can be reached only after a thorough analysis of the clinical situation, of the general status of the patient and following a clear definition of the aims of the treatment.

Moreover, these techniques must be concentrated in highly specialized institutions in order to avoid improper use, a dispersion of economic and human resources and an increase in morbidity and mortality in the treated patients.

This can be obtained only in a climate of open cooperation and in a highly scientific setting. In the light of our experience, here we briefly report on the rationale, technical aspects and clinical results of the most used locoregional therapeutic techniques in cancer which can be widely grouped into two main approaches: regional chemotherapy and image-guided tumor ablation.

Regional Chemotherapy

The theoretical basis of regional chemotherapy are based on the following hypotheses: (a) that this technique can deliver a high concentration of the antitumor agent to localized cancers and hence produce a higher response rate than in the systemic administration; and (b) that a significant amount of the drug will be removed after the first pass through the capillary bed of the target region and thus reduce the systemic drug availability and toxicity generated.

Tumors with minimal sensitivity to systemic chemotherapy might benefit from an incremental increase in a locally delivered drug dose. This is particularly true since most chemotherapeutic agents have a very steep dose-response curve.

The advantage of delivering drugs regionally by intra-arterial infusion depends upon the size of the artery infused, the rate of excretion of the agents used, the amount of the agent entering the tissue, especially from the first circulation, and the amount of the agent entering the tissue which is biologically active against tumor cells. Since total body clearance is inversely proportional to the area under the curve and principally to the toxicity of a chemotherapeutic agent, the rapidity of the clearance determines the usefulness of regional drug infusion.

The anti-metabolite FUDR used in treating colorectal cancer liver metastases is the only situation where a chemotherapeutic agent has a truly worthwhile regional advantage. This agent has a hepatic extraction ratio of approximately 92% and therefore the hepatic tumor drug exposure can be increased 100 to 400 fold. Five-FU, doxorubicin, mitomycin-C, nitrosourea and cisplatin are not as effectively cleared by the liver. In addition, because of the high regional blood flow (~1450 cc/min) within the liver, the tumor uptake of these agents is modest and their effectiveness on tumor response is minimal.

In 1967 Cavaliere reported the synergism of hyperthermia and high-dose chemotherapy in vitro. In 1975 Stehlin et al. reported the enhanced effects of chemotherapy in the presence of increased temperatures in humans. From this knowledge, hyperthermia has been introduced in most locoregional treatments.

At the same time a possible role of the locoregional approach was considered to treat neoplasms showing peritoneal dissemination. In the late 1970s, Dedrick described a model, based on physiological and anatomical characteristics of the peritoneal cavity as well as on previously reported pharmacokinetic data for some chemotherapeutic drugs, which suggested that the peritoneal cavity would be exposed to significantly more drug than the systemic circulation following the direct intraperitoneal administration of the agent. In this model the tumor in the peritoneal cavity might come into contact with much higher concentrations of drug than could be achieved with systemic delivery of the same agent.

At present there are three main procedures for delivering regional chemotherapy:
- Continuous infusion of drugs intra-arterially in a selected region
- Locoregional perfusion with extracorporeal circulation
- Intraperitoneal infusion/perfusion.

More recently, electrochemotherapy (ECT) has been introduced into clinical practice as a novel approach to drug delivery in cancer. ECT is based on electroporation, a physical delivery system to enhance the selective penetration of drugs, genes, or molecular probes into cancer cells by means of brief, externally applied electrical fields that increase cell membrane permeability.

Among several drugs tested in preclinical studies, bleomycin and cisplatin have been found to be the most suitable agents for this treatment approach.

Intra-arterial Infusion Chemotherapy for Liver Metastases

The only curative therapy for patients with isolated colorectal cancer liver metastases is hepatic metastasectomy. Unfortunately, most patients with liver metastases are not appropriate candidates for this option.

Most patients have tumors which cannot be removed either as a result of their size, number, location, or propinquity to major vessels or ducts within the liver. Although these patients are usually treated with systemic chemotherapy, those whose tumors are isolated to the liver are potential candidates for regional chemotherapy.

The locoregional delivery of chemotherapeutics to colorectal cancer liver metastases as a means to dose-intensify therapy has a sound anatomical basis. Unlike normal liver parenchyma, which is supplied predominantly by the portal vein, liver metastases derive their blood supply mainly from the hepatic artery. Therefore, intrahepatic arterial infusion allows high concentrations of drugs to be delivered more selectively to hepatic tumors. Continuous infusion of FUDR for extended periods appears to be the optimal method of its delivery. This maintains drug levels for multiple cell cycles, producing a maximum anti-tumor effect.

Technique

Hepatic arterial chemotherapy usually is administered through hepatic artery catheters connected to a subcutaneous port or pump. These devices have proven to be safer and less cumbersome than percutaneous catheters. Implanted pumps have been found to be less likely to become occluded than percutaneously placed ones [1].

Operative placement of hepatic arterial catheters is performed through a generous right subcostal incision. Cholecystectomy is routinely performed to prevent drug-induced cholecystitis.

It is important to dissect out several centimetres of the common hepatic and proper hepatic arteries so that all branches to the proximal duodenum and the gastric antrum can be ligated and divided. This is required to prevent the development of chemotherapy-induced gastritis.

Before placing the catheter into the gastroduodenal artery, a subcutaneous pocket is created over the right lower quadrant of the abdomen into which the pump port is placed and secured with proline sutures.

A small arteriotomy is made in the gastroduodenal artery, after the common hepatic artery and proper artery have been occluded with vessel loops or vascular clamps. The catheter is secured in this position with silk ties placed around the gastroduodenal artery just proximal and distal to each bead.

Clinical Results

Hepatic arterial infusion (HAI) may be offered to patients with unresectable liver metastasis in the absence of extra-hepatic disease. However, the efficacy of these treatments is still being determined [4]. Both systemic and locoregional chemotherapy might be useful in the neoadjuvant setting to increase the resectability of liver metastases initially not amenable to surgical resection. Even in previously treated patients, high response rates (73–88%) can be achieved with the association of HAI and systemic therapy and 23–35% of these patients were able to undergo liver resection.

The main toxicity from HAI FUDR is to the bile ducts rather than the liver parenchyma (sclerosing cholangitis). However, the toxicity appears after multiple treatments, usually after a clinically relevant tumor response. In fact, conversion to resectability may occur more quickly with HAI plus systemic therapy (60% at 2 months) versus systemic therapy alone [5,6].

Attempts have also been made to reduce the risk of relapse with either systemic adjuvant chemotherapy or chemotherapy and HAI after liver resection. Comparing standard systemic chemotherapy using 5-FU/leucovorin with alternating systemic therapy and HAI, patients receiving HAI showed lower risk of hepatic progression (23% vs. 68%), better 5-year survival (57% vs. 49%) and better median survival (37.4 vs. 17.2 months) [7]. In the light of the observed benefit, HAI is likely to potentiate the role of systemic chemotherapy in patients with inoperable liver metastases or as an adjuvant after resection.

Isolated Limb Perfusion

Isolated limb perfusion (ILP) was introduced for the treatment of patients with melanoma by Creech in 1957. The therapeutic efficacy of ILP for the treatment of locally recurrent melanoma and in-transit metastasis is well established as well for non-resectable limb sarcoma. ILP has undoubtedly led to improved local results with respect to those achieved with systemic therapy.

Technique

Depending on the location of the tumor, ILP can be carried out at several different levels. The perfusion level is chosen to achieve the smallest perfusion volume around the tumor, since this is associated with lower morbidity. The options for the upper limb are the subclavian, axillary and brachial arteries, while in the lower limb the external iliac, common femoral and popliteal arteries are used. At present, the most suitable drugs for ILP are melphalan (L-PAM) and tumor necrosis factor (TNF). L-PAM (10–13 mg/L of limb volume) is injected into the extracorporeal circuit at 38–41° C and the perfusion is carried out for 60 min. TNF-α is infused when temperature at the arterial level is 38.5° C. L-PAM is infused in the circuit 15–30 min later. Perfusion lasts 60–90 min from the time of infusion of TNF and the temperature is maintained at 38.5–40.5° C. At the end of ILP, the limb is washed with aprotin and 3,000–5,000 mL of saline solution for 5–7 min. Lastly, the vessels are sutured. Continuous leakage evaluation is carried out in patients receiving TNF-α by a nuclear medicine procedure.

Clinical Results

ILP with high-dose L-PAM currently produces good responses in most patients with locally advanced tumor. The toxicity of the procedure is primarily regional and consists of edema, erythema, and blistering as well as rare neuropathies or vascular complications and is generally classified by the Wieberdink scale. The reported amputation rate due to toxicity is 0.5–1% (Table 11.1). Systemic toxicity is limited, consisting of immediate postoperative nausea and vomiting and sometimes transient bone marrow depression often caused by a high leakage rate.

Results from the literature show a tumor response ranging between 7 and 77% in melanoma patients treated by ILP with L-PAM [8]. The different characteristics of the patients (number of lesions, nodal involvement and relapses) and the treatment employed (tumor temperature level and drug) provide a logical explanation for the heterogeneous results obtained. The addition of TNF-α at doses up to 10 times the maximum tolerable dose with or without interferon-γ (IFN-γ) allows a higher response rates (>80%) for locally advanced (bulky) melanoma [9–11].

With regards to sarcoma patients, it is questionable whether extensive surgery such as amputation or disarticulation is indicated in patients at high risk of general metastases and poor survival, while a locoregional approach could provide optimal local control (Table 11.2). Overall, patients who have undergone neoadjuvant ILP with L-PAM/doxorubicin + TNF-α show a limb sparing rate of nearly 80%. Overall, after tumor surgical excision, a long-term local control rate of 70% with a 5-year survival of 40% has been reported [12–15].

Table 11.1 Tumor response and toxicity after TNF-based isolated limb perfusion in sarcoma patients

Group	Patients		Response		Toxicity	
	No.	C	P	NC + PD	Local	Systemic
Eggermont 1996 [12] [12]	186	29	53	17	7.5(G4) 0.5(G5)	0.5–9.0 (G3–G4)
Gutman 1997 [14]	35	37	54	9	10(G4) 2 (G5)	0 (G3–G4)
Noorda 2003 [13]	49	8	55	37	25 (G3) 2 (G4)	– –
Cherix 2008	51	25	42	28	21 (G3) 2 (G5)	6 (G2) –
Rossi 2008 (unpublished data)	54	27	65	8	15 (G4) 0 (G5)	5 (G3) 0 (G4)

C, complete; *NC+PD*, no chance + progressive disease; *P*, partial

Table 11.2 Limb sparing and local control after TNF-based isolated limb perfusion in sarcoma patients

| Group | Patients | Conservative surgery | | Local control | |
		LSS (%)	Secondary amputation (%)	LRR (%)	Median F–U (mos)
Eggermont 1996 [12]	186	82	2	11	22
Gutman 1997 [14]	28	85	0	18	14
Noorda 2003 [13]	49	84	10	13	26
Cherix 2008	51	6	10	35	20
Rossi 2008 (unpublished data)	54	83	10	12	32

F-U, follow-up; *LRR*, local recurrence rate; *LSS*, limb-sparing surgery

Intraperitoneal Chemotherapy

Intraperitoneal chemotherapy (IPC) is based on a strong scientific rationale and is currently a fascinating area of research.

The theory concerning the peritoneal plasma barrier is based on different studies confirming the existing peritoneal-plasmatic gradient (20–600). The barrier, represented by the submesothelial tissue and the capillary basement membrane, limits the re-absorption of high weight and hydrophilic drugs such as mitomycin-C and cisplatin. The result is a longer permanence of drugs in the peritoneal cavity. The hyperthermic effects on drug activity are known to be related with: (a) increase in drug concentration; (b) drug activation process; (c) intracellular alkylating index; and (d) the inhibition of DNA repairing process.

Probably the major factor determining the limitations of intraperitoneal therapy is the depth of penetration of cytotoxic agents into the tumor, ranging from several cell layers to 1–3 mm from the tumor surface. This means that the superiority of intraperitoneal drug administration over intravenous delivery will be limited to those patients with very small tumor volumes when intraperitoneal treatment is initiated.

Another factor to consider is the dose-limiting toxicities of intraperitoneal drug administration either systemic and local. However, the clearance of IPC is lower than the plasma one and this is an important feature for locoregional treatment.

The major cause for limited effectiveness of cancer chemotherapy may be the amount of tumor burden. One strategy for minimizing treatment failure involves dose intensive regimens administered to patients with an absolute minimum tumor burden. To reduce tumor burden, cytoreductive surgery (CRS) is indicated.

Cytoreductive Surgery and Intraperitoneal Chemotherapy

Overall, the rationale to combine CRS and IPC is based on the following considerations:

- The resection site and abraded peritoneal surfaces are at high risk for tumor cell implantation in the postoperative period
- All intra-abdominal surfaces are fully exposed to IPC if the surgeon has been careful to separate all adherent structures and if these treatments are instituted prior to the formation of abdominal adhesions
- Regional chemotherapy may result in increased local responses without compromising systemic effects.

Technique

CRS means the complete removal of all macroscopic tumor in the peritoneal cavity. It could require peritonectomy procedures eventually associated with intestinal and/or organ resections. After surgery, the abdomen is lavaged clear of blood, blood products and tissue debris using large volumes of a peritoneal dialysis solution. Chemotherapy instillations are then performed on postoperative days 1–5 or 1–6 by means of intraoperatively positioned catheters.

Clinical Results

A meta-analysis of randomized trials of IP cisplatin in the initial chemotherapy treatment of ovarian cancer patients performed on six randomised trials of 1,716 patients showed that the pooled hazard ratio (HR) for PFS of IP cisplatin as compared to IV treatment regimens is 0.792 (95% CI: 0.688–0.912, $p= 0.001$), and the pooled HR for OS is 0.799 (95% CI: 0.702–0.910, $p=0.0007$). These findings strongly support the incorporation of an IP cisplatin regimen to improve survival in the front-line treatment of stage III, optimally debulked ovarian cancer [16]. However, further clinical trials are needed to determine the optimal drug for IP and optimal number of IP administrations in order to improve the survival rate in patients with advanced ovarian cancer [17].

To assess the efficacy and safety of IPC in patients undergoing curative resection for gastric cancer, eleven trials involving 1,161 cases were examined. The pooled odds ratio was 0.51, with a 95% confidence interval (0.40–0.65) in favor of patients having undergone IPC [18]. It was suggested that IPC may benefit the patients after curative resection for locally advanced gastric cancer, but continuous multicentre, randomized, double blind, rigorously designed trials should be conducted to draw definitive conclusions.

Cytoreductive Surgery and Hyperthermic Intraperitoneal Chemotherapy

Hyperthermic intraperitoneal chemotherapy (HIPEC) is the natural evolution of the IPC which diffusely developed during the last 3 decades. HIPEC is able to overcome some common limitations of IPC such as low drug penetration (no more than 1–3 mm in normothermic condition), limited diffusion due to the post-operative adhesions and relative local toxicity. HIPEC is an intra-operative approach that represents the synthesis of three different characteristics: the added efficacy of hyperthermia (more penetration into the tumor), the fluid dynamics of the system (better diffusion into the peritoneal cavity) and lastly the mechanical filtration process (elimination of microscopic cancer residual by filter).

Technique

HIPEC can be performed by open and closed abdomen techniques.

Open Abdomen

After completion of CRS, self-retaining Thompson retractors are positioned at the skin edges of the abdominal wound and suspended with running suture to the retractor frame. Two inflow catheters are placed respectively in the right subphrenic cavity, and at the deep pelvic level two outflow catheters are placed in the left subphrenic cavity and superficial pelvic site. The drains are connected with the extracorporeal circuit. At least two temperature probes are secured near the tip of the in-flow catheter and in the pelvis. Continuous peritoneal monitoring of temperatures during HIPEC is obtained by thermocouples placed in the abdominal cavity and subperitoneal site. The wound is covered by a plastic sheath sutured to the skin edges. Once the catheters are connected with an extracorporeal circuit a preheated polysaline is infused into the peritoneal cavity using a heart-lung pump at a mean flow of 600 mL/min. Normally 3–4 L of perfusate are used for the open abdomen technique and 5–6 L for the closed abdomen technique. After achieving the true hyperthermic phase (42.5° C), the drugs are injected into the circuit inflow line. The drug regimen is chosen according to the tumor histotype and the schedule of treatment, mitomycin-C and cisplatin being the drugs so far most used.

Following perfusion, the perfusate is quickly drained, the anastomoses performed and the abdomen closed after careful intraperitoneal observation.

Closed Abdomen

Before closing the abdominal wall after CRS, four silicone catheters are placed in the abdominal cavity through the abdominal wall. After closure of the abdominal skin the catheters are connected with the extracorporeal circuit. HIPEC is administered as reported above. Following perfusion, the abdomen is re-opened and anastomoses are performed.

Clinical results

The results of clinical trials on CRS and HIPEC in patients with peritoneal carcinomatosis from different types of cancer were recently reviewed and discussed during the 5th International Workshop on Peritoneal Surface Malignancy, held in Milan in 2006, aimed at creating a consensus. Overall, severe morbidity and mortality rates after CRS + HIPEC are not considered much higher than the 11% reported for CRS alone.

Taking into consideration the impact of CRS and HIPEC on patient survival, this multimodal therapeutic approach is currently considered beneficial for pseudomyxoma peritonei; the 5-year survival rate ranges between 52 and 72% [19]. Moreover, recent reports on peritoneal mesothelioma show that median survival after aggressive surgery combined with HIPEC has approached 5 years [20].

Analysis of evidence indicates prolongation of survival and potential for cure in patients with low volume metastatic adenocarcinoma of colonic origin limited to the peritoneal cavity too. However, in absence of a large prospective randomized trial, it is going to be difficult to demonstrate the true impact of CRS and HIPEC on the natural history of colorectal cancer with peritoneal dissemination [21].

The need for large multicentre randomized trials to confirm the benefits and risks of CRS associated with HIPEC is also advocated for patients with peritoneal carcinomatosis from gastric and ovarian cancers [22,23].

Electrochemotherapy

Nowadays, ECT has become a routinely used treatment modality and is a reliable treatment option for patients affected by cutaneous or subcutaneous metastasis not suitable for or not responsive to conventional therapies [24]. ECT allows high local tumor response rate with chemotherapeutic doses that by themselves cause no relevant side effects. Moreover, ECT is generally performed on an outpatient basis and has proven to be particularly useful in a palliative strategy in patients with in-transit metastases from melanoma but also with tumor nodules of different cancer histotypes [25].

Technique

The treatment is performed under local anesthesia or general sedation. Chemotherapeutic drugs (bleomycin or cisplatin) are administered either intravenously (bleomycin) or intratumorally (bleomycin or cisplatin) at a dose dependent on the body surface area or the size of the tumor nodules. Electric pulses are delivered by means of two types of needle electrodes (parallel arrays and hexagonal arrays) or a plate electrode is connected to a dedicated pulse generator.

Clinical Results

The European Standard Operating Procedure on Electrochemotherapy (ESOPE) study recruited 41 patients with cutaneous and subcutaneous nodules <3 cm in size. ECT proved to be effective both in melanoma and non-melanoma tumor nodules with a complete response in 74% of tumors, a partial response in 11%, and no change in 10% according to World Health Organization criteria; the local tumor control rate was 73 to 88% at 5 months after treatment [25]. In more recent clinical experiences, ECT proved to be safe, effective in different tumor types, and useful in preserving patient quality of life in a palliative setting [26].

Image-guided Tumor Ablation

As in the scheme of locoregional therapies reported above, a more detailed illustration of the techniques that determine the immediate destruction of tumor nodules using chemical or physical approaches will be presented as already standardized in the literature [27].

Main Techniques for Image-guided Tumor Ablation

The term tumor ablation is defined as the direct application of chemical or thermal therapies to a specific focal tumor (or tumors) in an attempt to achieve eradication or substantial tumor destruction. These procedures are more often performed percutaneously, but they can also be performed at laparoscopy, endoscopy or surgery. Nevertheless, given that image guidance is critical to the success of these therapies, most are performed by using a host of imaging modalities (i.e., fluoroscopy, ultrasonography (US), computed tomography (CT) and magnetic resonance imaging (MRI).

The methods of tumor ablation most commonly used in current practice are divided into two main categories: chemical ablation and thermal ablation. Chemical ablations are classified on the basis of the chemical nomenclature of the agent, such as ethanol and acetic acid, which induce coagulation necrosis and cause tumor ablation. Thermal ablation includes energy sources which destroy a tumor by using thermal energy, with either heat or cold. To date, the techniques mainly applied for thermal ablation are radiofrequency ablation (RFA), laser ablation (not covered here due to our limited specific experience), microwave ablation and cryoablation.

Radiofrequency Ablation and Microwave Ablation

RFA applies to coagulation induction from all electromagnetic energy sources with frequencies less than 30 MHz, although most currently available devices function in the 375–500 kHz range. Most devices currently used are monopolar in that there is a single "active" electrode, with current dissipated at a return-grounding pad. Bipolar devices have two "active" electrode applicators, which are usually placed in proximity to achieve contiguous coagulation between the two electrodes. Additionally, many electrode modifications are now available, including internally cooled electrodes and multi-tined expandable electrodes.

Microwave ablation refers to all electromagnetic methods of inducing tumor destruction by using devices with frequencies of at least 900 MHz up to 30 GHz and has been more recently introduced in clinical practice. It offers several theoretical advantages in comparison to RFA, such as higher intratumoral temperatures, larger tumor ablation volumes, faster ablation times, ability to use multiple applicators, improved convection profile and less procedural pain. In addition, microwave ablation does not require the placement of grounding pads.

Cryoablation

This term is used to describe all methods of destroying tissue by means of the application of low-temperature freezing. Cryoablation is now performed by using a closed cryoprobe that is placed on or inside a tumor. In the two main types of systems, argon gas and either gas or liquid nitrogen are used. Temperatures should be measured during two or more freeze-thaw cycles (active or passive thawing). The freezing of tissue with rapid thawing leads to the disruption of cellular membranes; other cell death mechanisms include interrupting blood flow to the tissue, causing ischemia, and apoptosis.

Image guidance refers to procedures in which imaging techniques are used during the procedure. Imaging is used in five separate and distinct ways: planning, targeting, monitoring, controlling, and assessing treatment response. US, CT, MRI, and more recently positron emission tomography (PET), are used to determine whether patients are suitable candidates for ablation. Imaging aspects that are particularly important include tumor size and shape, number, and location within the organ relative to blood vessels, as well as critical structures that might be at risk for injury during an ablative procedure. Targeting, monitoring, and controlling are all performed during the procedure, while the assessment of treatment response occurs after the procedure is completed and during follow up. In particular, real-time imaging modalities with multi-planar and interactive capabilities (for example, US, including contrast enhanced US, and some updated CT or MR imaging systems) are very useful during the placement of an applicator (e.g., an RF electrode or cryoprobe) and in monitoring how well the tumor is being covered by the ablation zone and whether any adjacent normal structures are being affected at the same time.

Indications and Results for the Ablation of the Principal Tumors

Image-guided ablation is most commonly used in the liver, but applications in pulmonary, renal and bone tumors are currently accepted. Regarding liver applications, ablation therapies were firstly used for treating hepatocellular carcinoma (HCC), followed by colorectal cancer liver metastases (CRCMTS).

Liver Tumors

Hepatocellular Carcinoma

According to both the European Association for the Study of the Liver and the American Association for the Study of Liver Diseases [28], percutaneous ablation is recommended as a curative treatment for non-surgical patients with "early" HCC (more recent studies, including randomized controlled trials, demonstrated image-guided ablation as effective as resection in cirrhotic patients). Particularly, alcohol injection and RFA are equally effective for tumors <2 cm; however, the necrotic effect of radiofrequency is more predictable in all tumor sizes and, in addition, its efficacy is clearly superior to that of alcohol injection in larger tumors. Also based on our experience [29], RFA is superior to alcohol injection in local control of early HCC (RFA should be the best choice in patients suffering from a more advanced oncological stage, such as a single lesion larger than 20 mm or multiple lesions), but this better performance does not necessarily translate into survival advantage for cirrhotic patients, mostly depending on liver function.

Moreover, RFA combined with TACE can also be useful in patients with non-early HCC, providing a relatively high complete local response (especially in lesions less than 5 cm in diameter) and promising midterm clinical success [30].

Colorectal Cancer Liver Metastases

In the last decade, percutaneous RFA has been widely used in the multimodal therapy of CRCMTS, although its clinical efficacy has not been clearly demonstrated due to the lack of randomized controlled trials. However, on the basis of several retrospective studies (considering predictors for technique safety and effectiveness, and survival), RFA and other ablation therapies (e.g. laser ablation, microwave ablation, etc.) can play a role in the case of unresectable CRCMTS. In our published series [31], as in others in the literature, we showed that small metastatic size favorably predicts survival. In fact, in unresectable patients, if there is no local success with RFA, other subsequent therapies would then be unable to stop disease progression. On the other hand, we reported that RFA was safer when not combined with vascular occlusion, which was initially adopted to enlarge the ablation zone and reduce local recurrence. Updated RFA devices or other energy source (i.e., microwaves) are now available to ablate the tissue surrounding the metastasis more widely and successfully treat nodules larger than 3 cm.

Finally, ablation therapies (either RFA or cryoablation) are frequently used as an effective adjunct to resection in achieving complete tumor clearance of the liver in patients in which surgery alone is unable to achieve an R0 resection.

11

Other Tumors

Lung

Although the number of reports on lung tumor ablation with different energy sources is progressively increasing, percutaneous RFA is the only well experimented technique for primary or metastatic nodules in non-surgical patients. In a large multicentre clinical trial, RFA yielded high proportions of sustained complete responses in properly selected patients with pulmonary malignancies, and was associated with acceptable morbidity [32]. However, before image-guided ablation becomes the choice therapy for unresectable lung tumors, randomized controlled trials comparing it with standard non-surgical treatment options (i.e., radiotherapy and systemic chemotherapy) are needed.

Kidney

The most frequently applied ablative techniques for low-grade renal cell carcinoma up to 4 cm in diameter are cryoablation and RFA. Urologists preferably use the former during laparoscopy, while radiologists usually perform the latter with a percutaneous approach under imaging guidance. However, interventional radiologists can choose their preferred technique taking into account personal experience and available equipment (percutaneous cryoablation or RFA; US, CT or MRI guidance) [33].

Safety and technique effectiveness of the two methods are much the same in the published series. In addition, considering predictors for local success and complications, percutaneous RFA can be proposed for non-central renal tumors up to 3 cm also in patients without surgical contraindications, thanks to comparable efficacy and favorable incidence of complications and costs in comparison to nephron-sparing surgical resection. Therefore, randomized controlled trials investigating long-term results of image-guided ablation versus surgery should be performed [34].

Bone

Few options are available for pain relief in patients with bone metastases who fail standard treatments. A multicentre study demonstrated that RFA provides effective palliation (significant pain relief) for cancer patients with localized painful osteolytic metastases involving bone, when they have failed standard treatments [35].

References

1. Ensminger WD (2001) Intraarterial therapy. In: Perry CM (ed) The chemotherapy source book, 3rd edn. Lippincott Williams & Wilkins, Philadelphia, pp 163–174
2. Rossi CR, Foletto M, Pilati P et al (2002) Isolated limb perfusion in locally advanced cutaneous melanoma. Semin Oncol 29:400–409

3. Markman M (1998) Intraperitoneal therapy in ovarian cancer. Semin Oncol 25:356–360
4. Alexander HR, Kemeny NE, Lawrence TS (2005) Metastatic cancer to the liver. In: De Vita VT, Hellmann S, Rosenberg SA (eds) Cancer principles & practice of oncology, 7th edn. Lippincott Williams & Wilkins, Philadelphia, pp 2352–2367
5. Lise M, Pilati P, Da Pian P et al (2003) Treatment options for liver metastases from colorectal cancer. J Exp Clin Cancer Res 22:149–156
6. Kemeny N (2007) Presurgical chemotherapy in patients being considered for liver resection. Oncologist 12:825–839
7. Vadeyar HJ (2007) Current therapeutic options for colorectal liver metastases. Indian J Gastroenterol 26:26–29
8. Rossi CR, Foletto M, Pilati P et al (2002) Isolated limb perfusion in locally advanced cutaneous melanoma. Semin Oncol 29:400–409
9. Rossi CR, Foletto M, Mocellin S (2004) Hyperthermic isolated limb perfusion with low–dose tumor necrosis factor-alpha and melphalan for bulky in-transit melanoma metastases. Ann Surg Oncol 11:173–177
10. Di Filippo F, Rossi CR, Santinami M et al (2006) Hyperthermic isolation limb perfusion with TNFalpha in the treatment of in-transit melanoma metastasis. In Vivo 20:739–742
11. Hayes AJ, Neuhaus SJ, Clark MA, Thomas JM (2007) Isolated limb perfusion with melphalan and tumor necrosis factor alpha for advanced melanoma and soft-tissue sarcoma. Ann Surg Oncol 14:230–238
12. Eggermont AM, Schraffordt Koops H, Klausner JM et al (1996) Isolated limb perfusion with tumor necrosis factor and melphalan for limb salvage in 186 patients with locally advanced soft tissue extremity sarcomas. The cumulative multicenter European experience. Ann Surg 224:756–764
13. Noorda EM, Vrouenraets BC, Nieweg OE et al (2003) Isolated limb perfusion with tumor necrosis factor-alpha and melphalan for patients with unresectable soft tissue sarcoma of the extremities. Cancer 98:1483–1490
14. Gutman M, Inbar M, Lev-Shlush D et al (1997) High dose tumor necrosis factor-alpha and melphalan administered via isolated limb perfusion for advanced limb soft tissue sarcoma results in a >90% response rate and limb preservation. Cancer 79:1129–1137
15. Cherix S, Speiser M, Matter M et al (2008) Isolated limb perfusion with tumor necrosis factor and melphalan for non-resectable soft tissue sarcomas: long-term results on efficacy and limb salvage in a selected group of patients. J Surg Oncol 98:148–155
16. Hess LM, Benham-Hutchins M, Herzog TJ et al (2007) A meta-analysis of the efficacy of intraperitoneal cisplatin for the front-line treatment of ovarian cancer. Int J Gynecol Cancer 17:561–570
17. Noma J, Yoshida N (2008) Intraperitoneal chemotherapy for ovarian cancer. Gan To Kagaku Ryoho 35:885–890
18. Xu DZ, Zhan YQ, Sun XW et al (2004) Meta-analysis of intraperitoneal chemotherapy for gastric cancer. World J Gastroenterol 10):2727–2730
19. Moran B, Baratti D, Yan TD et al (2008) Consensus statement on the loco-regional treatment of appendiceal mucinous neoplasms with peritoneal dissemination (pseudomyxoma peritonei). J Surg Oncol 98:277–282
20. Deraco M, Bartlett D, Kusamura S, Baratti D (2008) Consensus statement on peritoneal mesothelioma. J Surg Oncol 98:268–272
21. Esquivel J, Elias D, Baratti D et al (2008) Consensus statement on the loco regional treatment of colorectal cancer with peritoneal dissemination. J Surg Oncol 98:263–267
22. Helm CW, Bristow RE, Kusamura S et al (2008) Hyperthermic intraperitoneal chemotherapy with and without cytoreductive surgery for epithelial ovarian cancer. J Surg Oncol 98:283–290

23. Bozzetti F, Yu W, Baratti D et al (2008) Locoregional treatment of peritoneal carcinomatosis from gastric cancer. J Surg Oncol 98:273–276

24. Mir LM, Orlowski S (1999) Mechanisms of electrochemotherapy. Adv Drug Del Rev 35:107–118

25. Marty M, Sersa G, Garbay JR et al (2006) Electrochemotherapy–An easy, highly effective and safe treatment of cutaneous and subcutaneous metastases: results of ESOPE study. EJC[Suppl] 4:3–13

26. Campana LG, Mocellin S, Basso M et al (2009) Bleomycin-based electrochemotherapy: clinical outcome from a single institution's experience with 52 patients. Ann Surg Oncol 16:191–199

27. Goldberg SN, Grassi CJ, Cardella JF et al (2005) Image-guided tumor ablation: standardization of terminology and reporting criteria. Radiology 235:728–739

28. Bruix J, Sherman M (2005) Management of hepatocellular carcinoma. Hepatology 42:1208–1236

29. Brunello F, Veltri A, Carucci P et al (2008) Radiofrequency ablation versus ethanol injection for early hepatocellular carcinoma: a randomized controlled trial. Scand J Gastroenterol 43:727–735

30. Veltri A, Moretto P, Doriguzzi A et al (2006) Radiofrequency thermal ablation (RFA) after transarterial chemoembolization (TACE) as a combined therapy for unresectable non-early hepatocellular carcinoma (HCC). Eur Radiol 16:661–669

31. Veltri A, Sacchetto P, Tosetti I et al (2008) Radiofrequency ablation of colorectal liver metastases: small size favorably predicts technique effectiveness and survival. Cardiovasc Intervent Radiol 31:948–956

32. Lencioni R, Crocetti L, Cioni R et al (2008) Response to radiofrequency ablation of pulmonary tumors: a prospective, intention-to-treat, multicentre clinical trial (the RAPTURE study). Lancet Oncol 9:621–628

33. Veltri A, Garetto I, Pagano E et al (2009) Percutaneous RF thermal ablation of renal tumors: is US guidance really less favorable than other imaging guidance techniques? Cardiovasc Intervent Radiol 32:76–85

34. Veltri A, Calvo A, Tosetti I et al (2006) Experiences in US-guided percutaneous radiofrequency ablation of 44 renal tumors in 31 patients: analysis of predictors for complications and technical success. Cardiovasc Intervent Radiol 29:811–818

35. Goetz MP, Callstrom MR, Charboneau JW et al (2004) Percutaneous image-guided radiofrequency ablation of painful metastases involving bone: a multicenter study. J Clin Oncol 22:300–306

Hemostatic Agents in Surgical Oncology

12

S. Sandrucci

A wide variety of hemostatic agents and sealants have been developed as surgical tools, of which the uses now range beyond their namesake. According to FDA regulations, an hemostatic agent is defined as a device intended to produce hemostasis by accelerating the clotting process of blood. Broadly these agents can be thought of as topical hemostats, fibrin sealants, matrix hemostats and fibrin-coated collagen patch.

Topical Hemostats

Conventional topical agents include gelatins, oxidized cellulose and microfibrillar collagen. Gelatin products involve porcine gelatin moulded into a sponge that adheres to bleeding sites and causes platelets to be caught in uniform pores, activating the clotting cascade. Shortcomings include an inability to tamponade bleeding as well as potential disruption of the clot when the sponge is removed. The oxidized cellulose forms a lattice for clot formation. Since it does not enhance the clotting process, patients with coagulopathy and compromized platelet function may not benefit from this product. Microfibrillar collagen, which stimulates the intrinsic coagulation cascade, is formed by processing purified bovine collagen into submicron sized microcrystals. It is available in many forms, including a powder and a non-woven web [1].

Fibrin Sealants

The real value of fibrin sealants lies in their unique physiological action, which mimics the stages of the blood coagulation process and wound healing. Fibrin

S. Sandrucci (⌧)
Surgical Oncology Unit, S. Giovanni Battista University Hospital, Turin, Italy

New Technologies in Surgical Oncology. Antonio Mussa (Ed.)
© Springer-Verlag Italia 2010

sealants are biocompatible; degradation and re-absorption of the resulting fibrin clot is achieved during normal wound healing. Fibrin sealants are derived mainly from plasma components; most commercially available products contain purified, virally inactivated human fibrinogen and thrombin, with different quantities of factor XIII, anti-fibrinolytic agents (such as aprotinin) and calcium chloride. The sealant may be applied with a needle, as a spray or using other devices or applications. When fibrinogen and thrombin are mixed (during the application of the sealant to the liver surface), the fibrinogen component is converted to fibrin monomers [2]. Polymerization of fibrin monomers results in the formation of a semi-rigid fibrin clot which is capable of interacting with tissue structures. These interactions are essential for stimulating adherence of fibroblasts and their normal growth into the clot, in addition to well-oriented cell growth. By mimicking the later stages of the physiological coagulation system, these processes allow fibrin sealants to arrest blood loss and assist the wound healing process. Because fibrin sealants contain naturally occurring blood components, they produce clots which are hemostatic and can be degraded by the body's own fibrinolytic mechanisms within a few weeks. While the composition of most fibrin sealants is similar, different formulations and varying concentrations of key components, such as factor XIII, cause variation in the properties of the clots which are formed. Parameters such as speed of clot formation, adhesive strength and durability of the clot may be affected. Many factors, including the concentration of fibrinogen and thrombin, the presence of other plasma proteins, calcium concentration, ionic strength and temperature affect the rate and extent of fibrin polymerization and, ultimately, the structure of the clot.

Matrix Hemostats

FloSeal®, which was approved in December 1999, involves a proprietary gelatin matrix from bovine collagen which consists of microgranules cross-linked with glutaraldehyde [2]. Thrombin is mixed before use. As blood percolates through the matrix in the presence of bleeding, the granules swell approximately 20% within 10 min upon contact with blood, conforming to the shape of the wound and forming fibrin polymer. Clotting is enhanced with exposure to thrombin and the granules provide a framework for clot development. Human thrombin recently received FDA approval for pre-packaging. The long preparation time of fibrin sealant requires premixing components long before use. Therefore, the decision to use fibrin sealant must be made well before the necessity of its use can be established, i.e., uncontrolled hemorrhage. In addition, the fibrin sealant is difficult to inject if not used within 2–3 min of mixing in laparoscopic cases [3]. Gelatin matrix is used best as a pure hemostatic agent and not as a tissue glue or sealant.

Fibrin-Coated Collagen Patch

The combined use of a collagen patch and fibrin sealants is more effective than either agent alone for local hemostasis and tissue sealing. Therefore, collagen preparations which could be coated manually with fibrin sealants became available. However, these methods were ineffective in handling and variable in their effect. As a result, a ready-to-use system composed of a combination of a collagen carrier substance and a fibrin sealant, also known as fibrinogen coated collagen patch (TachoComb1, Nycomed Arzneimittel, Germany) were developed for use [4] combining the hemostatic and adhesive properties of coagulation factors to promote rapid hemostasis with the mechanical stability of a collagen patch. As a result, these sealants stay firmly in place after being positioned at the application site and prevent potential rebleeding [5]. Other major advantages include the inhibition of post-surgical adhesions [6]. As a ready-to-use biological adhesive material, sealant patches (SP) addressed many of the deficiencies of earlier biological sealing methods, and has since proved to have clinical benefits over other standard supportive treatments in a range of surgical procedures [4,5,7]. Aprotinin, an anti-fibrinolytic protease inhibitor, was originally added to liquid fibrin sealants to prevent the premature lysis of the fibrin clot, especially under hyper-fibrinolytic conditions. The first generation SP (SP-1) was composed of equine collagen, human fibrinogen, bovine aprotinin and bovine thrombin. In the second generation SP (SP-2), bovine thrombin was replaced by human thrombin. Subsequently, comparative pre-clinical studies performed under normal, stressful and hyper-fibrinolytic conditions showed that aprotinin was not essential for therapeutic efficacy. As the function of SP with or without aprotinin was shown to be equal, a third generation SP (SP-3) was developed in which aprotinin was omitted. Hence, the step-wise development process from SP-2 (TachoComb H) to SP-3 (TachoSil) entailed the complete removal of bovine aprotinin from the collagen fleece. The coagulation factors in SPs are dissolved upon contact with fluid and form the last stage of the coagulation cascade. After successful tissue sealing, the fibrin clot is degraded by fibrinolysis and cellular phagocytosis [8] while the collagen patch is degraded by absorptive granulation tissue and converted into a pseudo-capsule of endogenous connective tissue [8,9].

Pre-Clinical Experience with Fibrin-Coated Collagen Patch

Traction tests to determine the extensibility and tensile strength of TachoSil, carried out in both dry and wet state, showed that the extensibility rate was prolonged in the wet state. Under wet conditions tensile strength was reduced by 71%, while extensibility was 2.5 times greater than in the native, dry state [4]. High extensibility allows for natural movement of tissues and organs, especially parenchymatous tissues that possess similar characteristics. The high extensibility is accompanied by excellent adhesive strength, significantly higher than that achieved with alternative hemostatic preparations.

Experiments conducted under increased intra-organ pressure, hyper-fibrinolytic conditions, or inhibition of blood coagulation, add to the investigation of functional properties of artificial tissue dressings. In these studies, time to hemostasis was a commonly used endpoint for hemostatic efficacy, while incidence or intensity of leakage, such as visible air leakage or measurable drainage, was used to evaluate the efficacy of tissue sealing. In contrast to clinical use, where TachoSil is indicated as a supportive treatment to augment standard surgical procedures such as suturing, stapling or argon beamer, the same was used as the sole mean of achieving hemostasis and tissue sealing in all animal model studies. Studies conducted under normal conditions comparing second and third generation SPs in sealing splenic and liver lesions in dogs showed that both products achieved complete hemostasis [3,8]. No evidence of secondary hemorrhage was seen at necropsy, 48 h after surgery to coincide with the period of highest risk for recurrent bleeding in clinical practice, or of change in blood count or blood coagulation. In a pig spleen lesion model subjected to greatly elevated intra-splenic pressure, application of the third generation SP-3 to the experimental splenic lesions proved to be as effective as the second generation SP-2 in achieving hemostasis and tissue sealing. In this model, acute hemostatic efficacy was assessed immediately after application to heavily bleeding, splenic lesions, with resistance to biodegradation and proteolysis as investigated 72 h later by increasing the intra-splenic pressure by ligation of the splenic veins and IV administration of adrenaline. Although histopathological results at necropsy showed slightly greater degradation of the fibrin clot of the third generation SP-3, hemostatic and sealing effects were nonetheless maintained.

Safety and Toxicity

Because of its similarity in composition to SP-2, separate toxicological studies were not necessary for SP-3. Therefore, based on data from earlier pre-clinical toxicological studies on SP-2, SP-3 can be expected to have a safety profile that is at least comparable to the second generation, SP-2. Pre-clinical toxicological studies on second-generation SP-2, in which acute systemic toxicity following intraperitoneal insertion into rats and dogs was the primary endpoint, showed that at above therapeutic doses (up to 1000 mg/kg; equivalent to approximately 2 patches per kg bodyweight) there was no evidence of adverse effects on body weight, food consumption, hematology, blood clotting, blood chemistry and organ weights. No gross post mortem or histopathological findings of toxicological importance were identified. Local tolerance to the second-generation SP-2, assessed over a 6-month period following intraperitoneal insertion into dogs, showed no consistent evidence of specific adverse local reactions at the application site. Immunologically mediated inflammatory reactions were considered most likely due to the effects of mechanical irritation and were not considered a result of toxicity. Results from these studies show that SP-2, and by implication SP-3, is a very well tolerated preparation at doses 50–100 times the clinical dose for humans. Certainly, histopathological examination of tissues at necropsy in the various in vivo bridging studies showed no evidence of adverse local reactions to SP-3. In the pig spleen lesion model under greatly elevated intra-splenic pressure, for example, no excessive local reaction was detected even when the collagen fleece was in contact with the splenic vessels (gastrosplenic or hepatogastric). The lack of local and systemic toxicity is consistent with a product that is made from biodegradable materials, with good tissue histocompatibility, and one that is reabsorbed within a few weeks of application to target tissue [4].

Clinical Applications of Fibrin-Coated Collagen Patch in Surgical Oncology

The great advantage of fibrin-coated collagen patch is its ability to achieve hemostasis in critical conditions, thus minimizing the trauma on tissues and the need of applying blind stitches. The fact that it is a ready-to-use device makes its employ immediate and effective in critical conditions (Fig. 12.1).

Delgado et al. [10] evaluated the efficacy of a biological hemostatic fibrin patch to control coagulopathic bleeding and prevent death in a porcine model of severe liver injury. The ability of this dressing to effectively control and maintain hemostasis in this complex challenging model, especially when compared with hepatic packing, demonstrates that this product can serve as a novel hemorrhage control tool

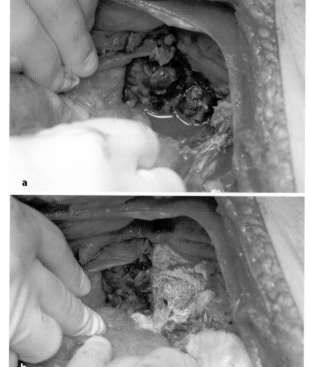

Fig. 12.1 After a debulking procedure of a pelvic mass (**a**), TachoSil is able to achieve optimal hemostasis without tissue trauma (**b**)

which could improve the outcome of patients with coagulopathic traumatic injuries both in civilian and military settings. After successful hemostasis the additional benefit of this re-absorbable dressing is that it could be left in a patient's body cavity after treatment, eliminating or reducing the need for additional surgery to remove hemostatic material. For the patient this could translate into a reduction in intensive care unit stay, rate of infection, morbidity, mortality, and overall cost.

Unfortunately there are no prospective trials in its use in surgical oncology; only several studies concerning specific applications have been reported.

Liver Surgery

While technical advances in liver surgery have made uncontrollable bleeding exceptional, postoperative mortality and morbidity are still related to postoperative bleeding, bile leakage and fluid accumulation – all potentially leading to repeated surgical or interventional treatment. Many methods and devices of dissection to skeletonize and subsequently control intra-parenchymal vessels and bile ducts have been introduced as a substitute for finger fracture of the parenchyma. In an effort to control diffuse oozing from the remaining surface of the transected liver and to complete biliostasis the use of fibrin based sealants has been advocated by many authors [11–14]. Control of bleeding from the parenchymal wound surface which affects postsurgical morbidity and mortality adversely remains a challenge in liver resection. Various techniques are used to reduce bleeding, and include ultrasonic or water-jet dissection, clamping of hepatic blood flow, argon beam coagulator and fibrin glues. There are few randomized clinical trials published with regard to the efficacy of fibrin glue in liver surgery – without comparison to argon beamer treatment [14]. Few controlled trials have been conducted to determine the comparative effectiveness of hemostatic agents in the control of diffuse bleeding of the raw surface of the liver; thus, treatment is often based on the surgeon's preference [11,12]. In a recent study TachoSil showed superiority over argon beamer with regard to the primary endpoint, time to hemostasis. This intraoperative endpoint is the "gold standard" for objective and measurable assessment of hemostatic efficacy of fibrin sealants and is recommended by the FDA. Most controlled trials of fibrin glues in liver resection have either no treatment or simple compression as comparator. Hemoglobin concentration of the drainage fluid proved to be significantly lower on day 2 in the TachoSil than in the argon beamer group. This was supported by a tendency towards lower hemoglobin concentration of the drainage fluid on day 1 in the TachoSil group. Interestingly, those results were obtained in spite of a larger mean size of target area for TachoSil (84 cm^2) than for argon beamer (65 cm^2), clearly indicating the more effective control of both intraoperative and postoperative bleeding from the resection surface by TachoSil. This may be due to the properties of TachoSil, which stabilize the local hemostatic effect, thus preventing any bleeding caused by postoperative hyper-fibrinolytic activity of cut or severed hepatic parenchyma [15].

The results of this study and of other multicentre, randomized studies [11,16] demonstrate that hemostatic agents are very effective in reducing the time required to achieve hemostasis following liver resection. Furthermore, they may lower the number of complications associated with liver surgery [16] and, consequently, provide high cost effectiveness.

Demirel [17] in an experimental setting has demonstrated that in liver surgery a higher incidence of abscess formation (33%) is observed if the hemostasis is achieved with a primary suture, while no abscess is observed if a fibrin-coated collagen patch is employed. This can be explained by the features of this technique which does not allow occurrence of any ischemic or blind areas or hematoma formation, as the fibrin sealant generates a quick and permanent sealing on blood and lymphatic veins by stopping fibrin exudation. According to a recent study, autologous fibrin gel possesses bactericidal properties in contaminated hepatic injuries [18]. Likewise, in a similar experimental study, the number of occurrences of abscesses was less extensive in the fibrin adhesive group than the suture group.

Elective Nephron-Sparing Surgery

Elective nephron sparing surgery is now an accepted standard of treatment for small, peripherally located kidney tumors. However, control of hemorrhage both during and after this type of surgery remains a challenge, with hemorrhage being a major complication. Hemostasis is especially important in urologic laparoscopy. The hemostatic efficacy and the safety of TachoSil in kidney resection surgery were clearly demonstrated by Siemer et al. [19]. The primary end point, time to hemostasis, showed TachoSil to be significantly superior to standard treatment for intraoperative control of hemorrhage from the parenchymatous wound following resection of the kidney. This result is supported by the finding that a significantly larger proportion of subjects in the TachoSil group obtained hemostasis within 10 min compared with the standard treatment group. The fact that approximately one third of standard treatment patients did not have bleeding controlled after 10 min has clinical relevance for the surgeon. The use of TachoSil as a local hemostatic thus seems a convenient method for the control of bleeding from the resection surface. Surgeons in the study rated TachoSil superior to standard treatment with regards to convenience of preparation, convenience of application, and impression of efficacy. These ratings confirmed the findings of the primary end point with regards to the hemostatic efficacy of TachoSil patch and highlighted its ease of use, most likely since it needs no preparation prior to application. The non-traumatic treatment with TachoSil may therefore potentially provide a valuable alternative to standard suturing in patients with only one kidney, where it becomes even more important to preserve kidney parenchyma.

Colon Surgery

Anastomotic leakage is a major complication which causes significant morbidity and mortality, especially in the early period of colonic anastomosis. None of the different surgical techniques has been found to be superior to another. However, routine use of fibrin glue or omental patch support has been recommended by some surgeons to improve colonic anastomotic security.

In an experimental study on rats [20], the colon was transected and then anatomized with sutures, sutures + fibrin-coated collagen patch or fibrin-coated collagen patch alone. Rats were sacrificed either 3 or 7 days after the anastomosis. Anastomoses were evaluated for perianastomotic adhesion formation, bursting pressures and histological features.

Fibrin-coated collagen patch was found to improve anastomotic integrity on postoperative day 3, but the bursting pressures when this patch was used were less than those after simple suture anastomosis on postoperative day 7. There was also no significant difference between the sutured and sutureless anastomoses covered with fibrin-coated collagen patch. Day 7 is the time when tissue collagen production is finalized and maturation of the healing process begins. The decreased bursting pressure during this period was unexpected as the main idea was to give additive strength with exogenous collagen. Van der Ham et al. [21] reported a reduced bursting pressure of rat colonic anastomosis 4 days after the operation when fibrin sealant was used. However, the pressures were observed to return to normal levels on postoperative day 7. Fibroblastic activity, collagen deposition and neovascularity were increased during normal healing when compared to anastomoses with the fibrin-coated collagen patch at postoperative day 7. In the early period of anastomotic healing, fibrin-coated collagen patch supports anastomotic integrity. However, it also causes an inflammatory reaction which may increase the time necessary for the healing process. This may be a major disadvantage for this biomaterial. As a consequence, its usage should be cautiously evaluated in clinical conditions and, if preferred in selective clinical cases, careful follow-up is mandatory.

Other Applications

Post-Axillary Lymph Node Dissection Seroma

Prolonged postsurgical drainage and lymphocele formation are significant complications after axillary lymph node dissection (ALND) for breast cancer. Lymphocele formation ranges from 3% to 50% in different series [22]. Known sequelae of these complications are increased rates of wound infection, dehiscence, and possibly delayed delivery of adjuvant therapy [23]. It can also cause minor problems, such as decreased mobility, arm swelling, poor cosmetic results, and prolonged hospitalization, which can be quite disturbing to the emotionally fragile, postsurgical breast cancer patient. The decrease in postsurgical drainage and early removal of the axillary drain would lead to early discharge from hospital, decreased postsurgical morbidity, and less discomfort to the patient. Different methods of preventing lymphocele formation and decreasing drainage after ALND have been used (i.e., surgical obliteration of axilla dead space, shoulder immobilization, or the use of pressure dressings), but none has proven to be beneficial. In this context, many investigators have evaluated fibrin glue as an adjunct to the conventional vacuum drain with conflicting results [24–28]. In a small series of 40 patients, Vaxman et al. prospectively evaluated fibrin glue in conjunction with a vacuum drain after axillary dissection for breast cancer and concluded that its use does not decrease postsurgical drainage. Furthermore, the rate of complication was significantly higher in the study group [24]. Ulusoy et al. prospectively studied 54 patients with breast cancer who underwent modified radical mastectomy. They found no benefit of the use of fibrin glue in postsurgical axillary drainage and no difference in lymphocele formation or wound infection was noted [25]. Dinsmore et al. reported on the effect of fibrin glue after modified radical mastectomy and found that its use increased time to drain removal as well as the complication rate. However, these differences did not reach statistical significance because of the small size of the series (27 patients) [26]. In a prospective, randomized study of 82 patients, Johnson et al. compared the use of fibrin glue with the use of Jackson–Pratt drain after several elective procedures for breast cancer (including simple mastectomy and SLND). No statistical difference was noted in lymphocele formation rate between the 2 groups; however, poor cosmetic results and extensive flap necrosis were noted in patients of the study group, which led to the withdrawal of 2 principal surgeons [27]. Moore et al. concluded that the use of fibrin glue decreased total drainage and time to drain removal [28]. In that study, the mean time to drain removal for lumpectomy patients was 14.8 ±9.6 days for the control group and 7.9 ±3.4 days for the study group (p <0.05). The period during which the drain was left in place for the control group was considerably longer than usual (14 vs. 7 to 8 days in the literature). All wound infections in this study occurred in fibrin glue-treated lumpectomy patients.

In a prospective, randomized, open, parallel-group, controlled clinical trial Berger et al. [29] evaluated the effect of a fibrin-glue coated collagen patch on volume and duration of postoperative axillary drainage, duration of hospital stay, and procedural safety. The authors observed no statistically significant differences with respect to axillary drainage time, drainage volume, length of hospital stay, local inflammation, and seroma formation after drainage removal.

Carless and Henry [30] conducted a systematic review of randomized controlled trials to examine the efficacy of fibrin sealants in reducing postoperative drainage and seroma formation after breast cancer surgery. Studies were identified by computer searches of Medline, Embase, the Cochrane Central Register of Controlled Trials and manufacturer websites and bibliographic searches of published articles. Trials were eligible for inclusion if they reported data on postoperative drainage and the number of patients who developed a seroma. The authors concluded that the current evidence does not support the use of fibrin sealant in breast cancer surgery to reduce postoperative drainage or seroma formation.

Therapeutic Inguino-femoral Lymph Node Dissection

Therapeutic inguino-femoral lymph node dissection (ILND) has been associated with clinically significant postoperative morbidities, including infections, skin flap compli-

12

cations, and lower extremity lymphedema, leading to extended hospitalizations, reduced quality of life, and delayed return to normal activities. A 50% incidence of complications following ILND in melanoma patients has been reported, and some studies have indicated that the incidence of short-term (within 30 days of surgery) and long-term morbidity from ILND may be as high as 75% [31,32]. Patients who have comorbidities that compromise their ability to walk, patients who have had complicated incisions for previous operations, obese patients, or patients who have locally advanced disease may experience even higher rates of postoperative morbidity. Despite these risks, therapeutic lymphadenectomy is generally performed for patients with confirmed node-positive stage III melanoma because it is the only potentially curative treatment. Currently, closed suction drains (CSDs) are inserted at the time of ILND to decrease seroma formation, wound dehiscence, and infection. However, CSDs are not without consequence: they require a high level of maintenance, cause discomfort, interfere with mobility, and serve as potential routes for infection when drainage is prolonged. Therefore, strategies which can be used to prevent postoperative fluid accumulation, thereby reducing the length of time CSDs are in place or even eliminating the use of the drains, potentially will decrease morbidity and increase the quality of life of patients undergoing ILND for melanoma. Mortenson [33] assessed the impact of CSDs and evaluated whether the intraoperative use of a fibrin sealant decreased time to drain removal and wound complications in melanoma patients undergoing inguino-femoral lymph node dissection. A single-institution, prospective trial was then performed in which patients were randomized to a group that received intraoperative application of a fibrin sealant following inguino-femoral lymph node dissection or to a control group that did not receive sealant. Postoperative closed suction drains were associated with major patient inconvenience. Applying a fibrin sealant at the time of inguino-femoral lymph node dissection in melanoma patients did not reduce the time to drain removal or postoperative morbidity.

References

1. Shekarriz B, Stoller ML (2002) The use of fibrin sealant in urology. J Urol 167: 1218
2. Carless PA, Anthony DM, Henry DA (2002) Systematic review of the use of fibrin sealant to minimize perioperative allogeneic blood transfusion. Br J Surg 89:695
3. Gill IS, Ramani AP, Spaliviero M et al (2005) Improved hemostasis during laparoscopic partial nephrectomy using gelatin matrix thrombin sealant. Urology 65:463
4. Schiele U, Kuntz G, Riegler A (1992) Hemostyptic preparations on the basis of collagen alone and as fixed combination with fibrin glue. Clin Mater 9:169–177
5. Hollaus P, Pridun N (1994) The use of tachocomb in thoracic surgery. J Cardiovasc Surg (Turin) 35[Suppl 1]:169–170
6. Osada H, Tanaka H, Fujii TK et al (1999) Clinical evaluation of a hemostatic and anti-adhesion preparation used to prevent post-surgical adhesion. J Int Med Res 27:247–252
7. Frilling A, Stavrou GA, Mischinger HJ et al (2005) Effectiveness of a new carrierbound fibrin sealant versus argon beamer as hemostatic agent during liver resection: A randomised prospective trial. Langenbecks Arch Surg 390:114–120

8. Schelling G, Block T, Gokel M et al (1988) Application of a fibrinogen-thrombin-collagen-based hemostyptic agent in experimental injuries of liver and spleen. J Trauma 28:472–475

9. Schneider A, Bennek J, Olsen KO et al (2006) Experimental study evaluating the effect of a barrier method on postoperative intraabdominal adhesions. Dig Dis Sci 51:566–570

10. Delgado AV, Kheirabadi BS, Fruchterman TM et al (2008) A novel biologic hemostatic dressing (fibrin patch) reduces blood loss and resuscitation volume and improves survival in hypothermic, coagulopathic swine with grade V liver injury. J Trauma 64:75–80

11. Chapman WC, Clavien PA, Fung J et al (2000) Effective control of hepatic bleeding with a novel collagen-based composite combined with autologous plasma: results of a randomized controlled trial. Arch Surg 10:1200–1205

12. Davidson BR, Brunett S, Javed MS et al (2000) Experimental study of a novel fibrin sealant for achieving hemostasis following partial hepatectomy. Br J Surg 87:790–795

13. Schenk WG, Burks SG, Gagne PJ et al (2003) Fibrin sealant improves hemostasis in peripheral vascular surgery: a randomized prospective trial. Ann Surg 6:871–876

14. Izbicki JR, Kreusser T, Meier M et al (1994) Fibrin-glue-coated collagen fleece in lung surgery. Experimental comparison with infrared coagulation and clinical experience. Thorac Cardiovasc Surg 5:306–309

15. Noun R, Elias D, Balladur P et al (1996) Fibrin glue effectiveness and tolerance after elective liver resection: a randomized trial. Hepatogastroenterology 43:221–224

16. Schwartz M, Madariaga J, Hirose R et al (2004) Comparison of a new fibrin sealant with standard topical hemostatic agents. Arch Surg 139:1148–1154

17. Demirel AH, Basar OT, Ongoren AU et al (2008) Effects of primary suture and fibrin sealant on hemostasis and liver regeneration in an experimental liver injury. World J Gastroenterol 14:81–84

18. Dulchavs.ky SA, Geller ER, Maurer J et al (1991) Autologous fibrin gel: bactericidal properties in contaminated hepatic injury. J Trauma 31:991–994; discussion 994–995

19. Siemer S, Lahmeb S, Altziebler S (2007) Efficacy and safety of TachoSil as hemostatic treatment versus standard suturing in kidney tumor resection: a randomised prospective study. Eur Urol 52:1156–1163

20. Ozel SK, Kazez A, Akpolat N (2006) Does a fibrin-collagen patch support early anastomotic healing in the colon? An experimental study. Tech Coloproctol 10:233–236

21. van der Ham AC, Kort WJ, Weijma M et al (1991) Effect of fibrin sealant on the healing colonic anastomosis in the rat. Br J Surg 78:49–53

22. Lumachi F, Brandes AA, Burelli P et al (2004) Lymphocele prevention following axillary dissection in patients with breast cancer by using ultrasound scissors: a prospective clinical study. Eur J Surg Oncol 30:526–530

23. Gonzalez EA, Saltzstein EC, Riedner CS et al (2003) Lymphocele formation following breast cancer surgery. Breast J 9:385–388

24. Vaxman F, Kolbe A, Stricher F et al (1995) Does fibrin glue improve drainage after axillary lymph node dissection? Prospective and randomized study in humans. Eur J Surg Res 27:346–352

25. Ulusoy AN, Polat C, Alvur M et al (2003) Effect of fibrin glue on lymphatic drainage and on drain removal time after modified radical mastectomy: a prospective randomized study. Breast J 9:393–396

26. Dinsmore RC, Harris JA, Gustafson RJ (2000) Effect of fibrin glue on lymphatic drainage after modified radical mastectomy: a prospective randomized trial. Am Surg 66:982–985

27. Johnson L, Cusick TE, Helmer SD et al (2005) Influence of fibrin glue on lymphocele formation after breast surgery. Am J Surg 189:319–323

28. Moore M, Burak WE Jr, Nelson E et al (2001) Fibrin sealant reduces the duration and amount of fluid drainage after axillary dissection: a randomized prospective clinical trial. J Am Coll Surg 192:591–599

12

29. Berger A, Tempfer C, Hartmann B et al (2001) Sealing of postoperative axillary leakage after axillary lymphadenectomy using a fibrin glue coated collagen patch: a prospective randomised study. Breast Cancer Res Treat 67:9–14

30. Carless PA, Henry DA (2006) Systematic review and meta-analysis of the use of fibrin sealant to prevent seroma formation after breast cancer surgery. Br J Surg 93:810–819

31. Tonouchi H, Ohmori Y, Kobayashi M et al (2004) Operative morbidity associated with groin dissections. Surg Today 34:413–418

32. de Vries M, Vonkeman WG, van Ginkel RJ et al (2006) Morbidity after inguinal sentinel lymph node biopsy and completion lymph node dissection in patients with cutaneous melanoma. Eur J Surg Oncol 32:785–789

33. Mortenson MM, Xing Y, Weaver S (2008) Fibrin sealant does not decrease seroma output or time to drain removal following inguino-femoral lymph node dissection in melanoma patients: A randomized controlled trial (NCT00506311). World J Surg Onc 6:63

Palliative Techniques and Supportive Procedures in Surgical Oncology

13

P. Racca, B. Mussa, R. Ferracini, D. Righi, L. Repetto, R. Spadi

Introduction

In palliative treatment surgery plays an important role: the primary aim of any palliative surgery is the relief of symptoms, with preservation or improvement in the quality of life [1]. In oncological practice, palliative surgery in the broadest sense refers to surgery that is by nature non curative. Palliative surgery also involves surgical procedures that are aimed primarily at the treatment of symptoms or complications associated with the tumor.

Symptom palliation is becoming a more important aspect in clinical trial evaluation and comprehensive care. In recent years an increasing numbers of articles have been published about the effects of cancer treatments on quality of life [2,3].

Palliative procedures and techniques have an important role to play in achieving pain and symptom relief. They include the formation of ostomies, the insertion of stents, paracentesis, orthopedic procedures such as spinal stabilization, the insertion of spinal catheters, radiotherapy and palliative chemotherapy.

Palliative care and the broader concept of supportive care involve the collaborative efforts of an interdisciplinary team. This team must include the discipline of medical, radiation and surgical oncology; orthopedics; urology; nursing; neurology and neuro-oncology; anesthesiology; psychiatry and psychology; pharmacology and many others [3].

P. Racca (✉)
Medical Oncology - C.U.R.O., S. Giovanni Battista University Hospital, Turin, Italy

New Technologies in Surgical Oncology. Antonio Mussa (Ed.)
© Springer-Verlag Italia 2010

Urogenital Problems

Progressing neoplasms can interfere with the urinary tract with dramatic progression of symptoms. Some inoperable kidney neoplasms may produce significant hemorrhagic events with associated anemia or major hypovolemic shock; blood inside the urinary tract could also clot and cause an occlusion, producing colic-like symptoms. In these cases renal artery embolization or polar artery embolization could be effective. Obviously this treatment is detrimental for the excretory function of the affected kidney, but the contralateral organ is often sufficient for sustaining life.

Retroperitoneal neoplasms, intra-abdominal tumor or lymphatic metastasis may compress the urinary tract or a renal vessel. Prostatic cancer or bladder cancer may stop urine flow due to stenosis or massive compression. This outcome could induce hydronephrosis with colic pain and often renal sepsis and associated septicemia and a general worsening of the condition [2].

Double J insertion can resolve these dramatic situations, allowing urine flow also in the presence of stricture or external compression and producing an immediate response to pain and renal failure. After the procedure mild urinary urgency and a little bleeding can occur but these symptoms regress in a few days. Double J insertion is performed with an endoscopic approach in local anesthesia. If stricture or compression cannot be overcome, a radiologic approach with percutaneous pyelostomy must be utilized to avoid damage of the urinary tract [4].

Penile neoplasms may also involve the urinary tract with obstruction. In these cases no trans-urethral approach can be used, so percutaneous cystostomy must be performed. This artificial window between the bladder and the skin is placed in the suprapubic area with a small tube to drain urine. As this device can also become obstructed it must be changed or cleaned every 2/3 months [3].

Biliary Obstruction

In biliary obstruction, interventional radiology is a bridge between diagnosis and therapy offering the best diagnostics and treatment of the disease using angiographic derived instruments [5–7]. Percutaneous treatment of biliary obstruction started in 1972 with the possibility of obtaining correct biliary duct imaging by percutaneous puncture of the biliary tract for diagnostic and therapeutic purposes. Local anesthesia and angiographic stents enable treatment in 90% of cases [6], even in critical patients.

Currently percutaneous cholangiography is performed only when therapeutic treatment is needed, because MR cholangiography is able to provide high quality images of the biliary tract for diagnostic purposes [7]. Percutaneous access to the biliary tract is obtained using a 21–22 G Chiba needle inserted under radioscopic guidance along the midaxillary line at the 10th or 11th costal space to avoid the costophrenic area [8]. During the procedure biopsy samples of the obstructive lesion can be taken if required. Complications are rare, but dramatic when they occur: hemoperitoneum, general sepsis or biliary peritonitis.

Biliary drainage is performed in malignant stenosis or obstruction and in postoperative fistula. It may be used as a permanent or temporary bridge to surgery, even with palliative intent. If stenosis or obstruction cannot be passed, a multi-hole tube is inserted as an external drain. In contrast, when the stricture or obstruction can be passed with a guidewire, a long multi-holed tube can be inserted, thus bridging the two parts of the biliary tract and enabling the physiological flow of bile to the duodenum [7].

After biliary drainage, a stent or endoprosthesis may be implanted or bilioplasty may be performed. This procedure consist of the dilatation of the obstructed duct by an angioplastic-like balloon catheter inserted over a metal wire. Balloon inflation provides good dilatation of even hard malignant stenoses. After the procedure an external-internal catheter is left in place for several days.

Plastic Endoprosthesis and Metallic Stent

Plastic endoprosthesis or metallic stent placement is preferred to surgical treatment with palliative intention because it is less invasive and can also be performed under local anesthesia. Currently stenoses of the lower biliary tree, such as periampullary stenosis, are preferentially approached by endoscopic treatment; intrahepatic or biliary tract stenosis are treated by a percutaneous approach [9].

Plastic endoprostheses are placed about 5-10 days after the drainage procedure. A protective drainage remains for some days to permit easy treatment of complications such as obstruction or bleeding.

Metallic stent placement is more effective for definitive treatment, due to the larger diameter of the device which is less prone to obstruction The main pitfall of metallic self-expandable stents is that the peculiar net structure firmly anchors the prosthesis to the stenosis, so that it cannot be changed or removed in the event of complications [9].

Mandatory indications for percutaneous treatment include contraindications to surgical treatment, preoperative treatment, endoscopic treatment failure, emergency, improvement in quality of life without impacting on life expectancy.

Relative contraindications include ascites, non-compliant patients, INR>2.5, hepatic vascular neoplasms or malformations, and known allergy to contrast material. Percutaneous drainage is absolutely contraindicated in patients with intrahepatic or confluence occlusion of the biliary tract with impossibility to drain a sufficient amount of liver parenchyma [10].

Complications

Mortality is near zero and complications of the percutaneous procedure rarely require surgical treatment. Major complications include biliary leakage requiring an additional interventional radiological procedure and major bleeding requiring intravascular embolization [11].

The most frequent complications are sepsis, which may develop after the procedure and not be responsive to antibiotic treatment. An antibiogram is mandatory in these cases and prevention can be achieved with drainage substitution every 2–3 months. Hemobilia may be venous or arterial. The former is not severe, but often and especially if the puncture is near the hepatic hilum they can be difficult to distinguish from one another, so an arteriography is needed and embolization is the right treatment.

Minor complications include [11]:

- Bile leakage from skin hole, due to a long lasting drainage or catheter occlusion. This is resolved by replacement with a larger gauge catheter
- Bilioma, due to incorrect alignment between the parietal and hepatic drainage hole. Infection may occur so drainage is mandatory
- Pain, due to possible compression of a costal nerve by the intercostal drainage transit. Symptoms usually spontaneously diminish within a few days, otherwise the insertion area must be changed
- Hyperamylasemia: a frequent temporary phenomenon and as such monitoring of pancreatic function in all patients undergoing the procedure is mandatory. Necrotic-hemorrhagic pancreatitis is otherwise quite rare.

Refractory Ascites

Ascites is a frequent symptom in patients with advanced abdominal neoplastic disease. Ascites can be primitive, i.e., when the peritoneum is involved by neoplastic diffusion, or secondary to liver dysfunction due to hepatic metastases or tumoral cachexia. International guidelines [12] show that medical management is mandatory before using invasive procedures. In this case diuretics, a low salt diet and in selected cases infusion of albumin are the mainstay of treatment. When the latter is not satisfactory drainage of the ascites is needed.

The first choice procedure must be performed with ultrasound guidance [13], to avoid intestinal or vascular damage, especially in a re-operated abdomen. Usually paracentesis is performed using a large gauge needle and in local anesthesia. Liquid must be examined for cytological and bacteriological studies. As the number of punctures increases, so too does risk and patient discomfort; in these cases, permanent drainage could be adopted to resolve this problem.

Drainage may be simple external, tunnelled external or peritoneum-jugular shunt. A simple external drainage is a silicon tube inserted with a small incision inside the abdominal cavity. Normally this procedure is performed at the end of a surgical procedure. In the case of ascites the exit hole must be small to avoid leakage around the tube. Usually a colostomy bag placed around the puncture site can prevent this problem. The technique is simple but requires abdominal insertion in the operating theatre, discomfort for the patient is high as is the risk of obstruction [13].

Tunnelled external drainage can be performed by open access or with a percutaneous approach [14]. In the first case at the end of the surgical procedure a cuffed tube for peritoneal dialysis is inserted into abdomen and tunnelled under the skin for 4–5 cm. This technique grants comfort to the patient and is safe, but requires a surgical approach to be completed. The other approach is percutaneous access obtained using a coaxial vascular catheter of 10–12 Fr inserted with a Seldinger maneuver under ultrasound guidance and tunnelled subcutaneously from the puncture site for almost 10 cm [12,14]. Coaxial catheters are generally made of soft polyurethane material and are well tolerated by the patient.

Peritoneal shunts have been used for patients with refractory ascites [15]. These allow continuous re-infusion of ascitic fluid from the peritoneal cavity via a one-way valve directly into the superior vena cava. Both LeVeen and Denver shunts have been developed and insertion allows a reduction in abdominal pressure and resolution of symptoms [15,16]. The objective of using these shunts is to achieve comfort and prevent the need for repeated paracentesis, thus avoiding massive protein loss. The procedure is associated with a number of complications such as shunt occlusion, infection, loculation and coagulation disorders. Despite this, it has been estimated to palliate symptoms effectively in approximately 70% of selected patients [15] and in the absence of contraindications, it would seem appropriate to consider this procedure in those patients who are expected to live long enough to derive benefit from it. The most frequent complication of shunting appears to be disseminated intravascular coagulation, although this is usually subclinical. Most authors have suggested that peritoneovenous shunting is associated with the risk of tumor dissemination from the peritoneal cavity to the pulmonary vessels [12]: while the theoretical risk of tumor dissemination exists, it is not clear if this is clinically significant. Complications are more frequent in those patients with positive cytology of ascitic fluid [12]. These include coagulopathy, infection and tumor embolization [16], suggesting that contraindications for shunt insertion should include pseudomyxoma peritonei, recent or current infection, preoperative coagulopathy, liver failure and loculated ascites. Relative contraindications include positive cytology in ascitic fluid and concurrent cardiac failure. Overall the mean functional shunt survival time is approximately 12 weeks [12,15,16].

Orthopedic Palliation

Important issues in oncology are both survival and quality of life of patients: both elements largely depend on tumor capability to produce metastasis. The most common sites of metastasis are the lung and bone. The latter may be complicated by vertebral fractures with nervous complications, skeletal fracture or impending skeletal fractures of the limbs, pain or hypercalcemia. Patients often need either hospitalization or they are bedridden. As such, the recently developed orthopedic oncology methods represent a fundamental stage in cancer patients treatment [17].

In recent years, treatment has been standardized with guidelines in many countries, e.g., Italian Guidelines by the Italian Society of Orthopaedics and Traumatology[18].

In addition to osteosynthesis techniques, mini-invasive palliative orthopedic surgery has also been recently developed, relying mainly on percutaneous methods. They are indicated when life expectancy is shorter than 1 year, when non-load bearing bones are affected, when lesions cause pain of a biological nature (infiltration), mechanical nature (bone insufficiency) and especially when radiotherapy is insufficient to resolve pain.

Osteosynthesis

Capanna and Campanacci classified the type of patient to be submitted to osteosynthesis according to a four stage system. Compared to traditional orthopedic indications, metastatic bone osteosynthesis provides immediate and survival-compatible stability [19].

Pathological fractures and impending fractures should always be treated. The risk of fracture can be evaluated by scores such as Mirel's, while recent finite element models coupled with CT scan have been proposed as a more precise method to define fracture risk.

Recently, computer assisted methods for osteosynthesis have been proposed. The advantages of these techniques include lower radiation exposure for both surgeons and patients and higher precision [18].

Mini-invasive Techniques: Radiofrequency Thermoablation

A 250-W instrument is usually applied for thermoablation, with continuous monitoring of the temperature provided and with 5 different electrodes applied to a StarBurst disposable applicator [20]. The instrument can be provided with 3 to 9 monopolar electrodes, opened to a sphere space pattern in order to obtain controlled tissue necrosis.

The technique can be performed within a CT scan gantry, with spinal or plexus anesthesia. The lesion is identified on the CT monitor and centred by a Kirschner wire, which is then substituted by a protection catheter. The StarBurst instrument is introduced through the protection catheter.

An international multicenter study in 2004 evaluated the method. Intermediate pain patients were included (from 7/10 up on a ten-point scale). The findings revealed that 95% of the treated patients gained a two-point pain reduction and reduced use of analgesics [20].

The method cannot be used in the following cases: less than 1 cm distance from noble structures such as the spinal cord and major nerve branches, major blood vessels (such as the aorta or vena cava), the bladder, etc. This technique does not replace osteosynthesis when indicated, rather it is an adjuvant treatment.

The other method for inducing percutaneous tumor necrosis is the use of radiofrequencies. The method again can induce the desired necrosis without obviously conferring any new mechanical strength upon the "healthy" bone. Therefore the indication for the radiofrequency technique includes those lesions which do not affect the mechanical competence of the affected bone [18].

Percutaneous Cementoplasty

Bone metastasis cementoplasty has been used as a fundamental step in open surgery after curettage of primary and secondary tumor lesions of bone. The acrylic cement fills the bony defect and confers mechanical stability to the osteolytic bone. Furthermore, cements polymerised with antibiotics or anti-blastic drugs can release the active compounds in the adjacent bone [21].

Cement can be introduced percutaneously into the bony lesion. This method acquired popularity for the treatment of vertebral somatic osteolysis and osteoporotic vertebral fractures. Somatic cementation of osteolytic lesions prevents fractures and avoids complications such as cord compression.

In the wake of the successful application of percutaneous vertebroplasty and its cement retaining variant kyphoplasty, cementoplasty has been proposed as an isolated technique for the percutaneous treatment of various localizations of bony lesions such as acetabular lesions [22], which is known as acetabuloplasty.

Reinforcement of the supra-acetabular anterior or posterior column is a complex operation using traditional open surgery synthesis and has few indications in the multiple metastatic patient. Conversely acetabuloplasty might be performed in combination with open treatment for osteolytic lesions or pathological fractures of the proximal femur [21]. Symptomatic relief after the procedure is obtained in the six-month postoperative period in a relevant percentage of cases, depending on the location and the extension of the osteolysis.

Absolute contraindications for percutaneous cementoplasty is the loss of cortical integrity of the bone where a leakage of the cement in the fluid phase might be responsible for soft tissue damage. It is therefore important to perform a CT bone scan for the study of the cortical bone adjacent to the lesion before performing the procedure. During the procedure it is often useful to obtain a tissue sample of the lytic area for staging or diagnostic purposes [18].

Medical Management

Malignant Bowel Obstruction

Patients with advanced-stage gastrointestinal malignancies can present bowel obstruction. The management of patients with obstruction secondary to widespread recurrence or carcinomatosis is a particularly challenging problem. When palliative surgery is not technically feasible or in patients with limited life expectancy, pharmacological management is indicated and is focused on the treatment of nausea, vomiting, pain and other symptoms.

A nasogastric tube (NGT) is useful for achieving decompression of the stomach or intestine, but it should be used only as a temporary measure because it is intrusive and distressing for the patients and may cause local complications. Pharmacological management principally consists of an association of anti-emetics (metoclopramide in patients with partial occlusion and no colic; haloperidol, cyclizine, prochlorperazine), anti-secretory drugs (hyoscine butylbromide, glycopyrrolate, octreotide) and analgesics [23]. Anti-emetics and analgesics should be used alone or in association with anti-secretory drugs to relieve symptoms, thus avoiding the placement of the NGT. The drugs of choice vary between countries and centres depending on personal clinical experiences, drug availability and costs. Vomiting may be controlled using anti-emetic drugs with a specific central effect or with anti-cholinergic drugs able to reduce gastrointestinal secretion. In recent years, steroids and somatostatin analogs have been successfully used as anti-secretory/anti-inflammatory drugs, according to the most up-to-date views of the pathophysiology of bowel obstruction. Clinical practice recommendations for the management of malignant bowel obstruction in patients with end-stage cancer have recently been published by the Working Group of the European Association for Palliative Care [23]. Parenteral hydration (intravenous or via hypodermoclysis) is sometimes indicated to correct nausea, whereas regular mouth care is the treatment of choice for dry mouth. Administration of 1–1.5 L/day of solution containing electrolytes and glucose may be useful in preventing symptoms due to metabolic derangement.

The route of drug administration depends on the clinical circumstances. In most obstructed patients oral administration is unreliable because of frequent vomiting. Rectal and sublingual medication are useful alternatives, particularly for patients being cared for at home. The transdermal route is available for administration of scopolamine and fentanyl. Where a pre-existing central venous line is not available, continuous subcutaneous infusions allows a constant infusion of medications over 24 h with minimum discomfort for the patient.

Dyspnea

There are several causes of dyspnea in cancer patients and many different mechanisms may coexist in a given patient. Cardiopulmonary causes are the main pathogenesis of dyspnea: parenchymal infiltration and malignant pleural effusion, lymphangitis, pericardial effusion and airway obstruction [24].

Although dyspnea in patients with advanced cancer is frequent and this symptom causes suffering, few controlled studies with an adequate number of patients have been carried out to study an adequate treatment. The role of oxygen therapy in reducing dyspnea in advanced cancer patients is still a controversial issue. In clinical practice it is possible to observe that in some cancer patients oxygen therapy can alleviate dyspnea unrelated to hypoxia.

In the case of cancer-related dyspnea, all the studies published to date have agreed on the beneficial effect of systemic opioids for cancer dyspnea [25]; however the optimal type, dose and modality of administration of opioids has not yet been established. Systemic opioids, by the oral or parenteral routes, can be used to manage dyspnea in advanced cancer patients. Nebulized morphine should not be used to treat dyspnea. A systematic review included a meta-analysis of nebulized opioids and systemic opioids for treating dyspnea and concluded that oral and parenteral opioids could be used to treat dyspnea ($p=0.0006$), while the use of nebulized opioids could not be supported ($p=0.31$).

Although benzodiazepines are commonly used in the symptomatic treatment of cancer-related dyspnea, no controlled clinical trials have been performed in cancer patients [24,25]. In some patients, benzodiazepines may be used when dyspnea is considered to be a somatic manifestation of a panic disorder or when patients have co-existent severe anxiety; however, both conditions are infrequent in patients with advanced cancer.

Bleeding

Hemorrhage occurs in approximately 6–10% of patients with advanced cancer. When visible, it can be particularly distressing to patients and their caregivers.

If the patient's goals of care are palliative, then management may include measures to stop the bleeding without full resuscitative measures. Comfort measures alone may be most appropriate for end-stage patients. The goals of care in a patient in the terminal phases of cancer should be comfort [26]. Invasive treatments may present more burden than benefit in these patients, and comfort without invasive procedures takes precedence. In some cases, it is unclear as to whether or not a local or systemic measure will be of more benefit. When a terminally ill patient is identified as being at risk for a major hemorrhage, family members and caregivers need to be sensitively informed and prepared, since these events can be extremely distressing. Using dark towels to absorb blood, applying pressure to the site of hemorrhaging, and placing patients in the lateral position (in the event of hematemesis or hemoptysis) are simple empowering measures. A rapid-acting sedative should be available for sedation; midazolam, 2.5 mg or 5 mg intravenously or subcutaneously, serves this purpose well.

References

1. World Health Organization (2002) National cancer control programmes: policies and managerial guidelines, 2nd edn. World Health Organization, Geneva
2. Doyle D, Hanks G, Nathan N, Calman K (2005) Oxford textbook of palliative medicine, 3rd edn. Oxford University Press, Oxford
3. Abrahm JL (2003) Update in palliative medicine and end-of-life care. Annu Rev Med 54:53–72
4. Patel U, Abubacker MZ (2004) Ureteral stent placement without postprocedural nephrotomy tube: experience in 41 patients. Radiology 230:435–442
5. Gandini G, De Ferrari F, Cassinis MC et al (2000) Radiologia Interventistica. Radiologia Forense 24:665–680

6. Righi D, Cassinis MC, Virzì V, Gandini G (2006) Patologia di fegato, vie biliari, pancreas: problematiche della radiologia interventistica. In: Guglielmi G, Schiavon F, Cammarota T (eds) Radiologia geriatrica. Springer-Verlag Italia, Milan, pp 397–403

7. Gandini G, Cassinis MC, Milanesio B et al (2003) Diagnostica e radiologia interventistica delle vie biliari. In: D'Amico D (ed) Nuovo trattato di tecnica chirurgica: fegato, vie biliari, asse spleno-portale. Utet, Turin, pp 342–345

8. Righi D, Bartoli G (2000) L'approccio transepatico all'albero biliare nella patologia ostruttiva. Hepatology Review 2:41–56

9. Tsuyuguchi T, Takada T, Miyazaki M et al (2008) Stenting and interventional radiology for obstructive jaundice in patients with unresectable biliary tract carcinomas. J Hepatobiliary Pancreat Surg 15:69–73

10. van Delden OM, Laméris JS (2008) Percutaneous drainage and stenting for palliation of malignant bile duct obstruction. Eur Radiol 18:448–456

11. Weber A, Gaa J, Rosca B et al (2008) Complications of percutaneous transhepatic biliary drainage in patients with dilated and nondilated intrahepatic bile ducts. Eur J Radiol [Epub ahead of print]

12. Becker G, Galandi B, Blum H (2006) Malignant ascites: systematic review and guideline for treatment. Eur J Cancer 42:589–97

13. Rosenberg S, Courtney A, Nemcek AA et al (2004) Comparison of percutaneous management techniques for recurrent malignant ascites. J Vasc Interv Radiol 15:1129–1131

14. Barnett TD, Rubins J (2004) Placement of a permanent tunneled peritoneal drainage catheter for palliation of malignant ascites: a simplified percutaneous approach. J Vasc Interv Radiol 15:379–383

15. Won JY, Choi SY, Ko H et al (2008) Percutaneous peritoneovenous shunt for treatment of refractory ascites. J Vasc Interv Radiol 19:1717–1722

16. Clara R, Righi D, Bortolini M et al (2004) Role of different techniques for the placement of Denver peritoneovenous shunt (PVS) in malignant ascites. Surg Laparosc Endosc Percutan Tech 14:222–225

17. American Cancer Society (2007) Cancer facts and figures. American Cancer Society, Atlanta

18. Società Italiana di Ortopedia e Traumatologia (2008) Linee guida SIOT per il trattamento delle metastasi ossee. www.siot.it

19. Capanna R, Campanacci DA (2001) Treatment of appendicular metastasis. J Bone Joint Surg 83:471–481

20. Albisinni U, Rimondi E, Bianchi G et al (2004) Experience of the Rizzoli Insitute in radiofrequency thermal ablation of musculuskeletal lesions. J Chemother 16 (Suppl 5):75–78

21. Cotten A, Deprez X, Migaud H et al (1995) Malignant acetabular osteolyses: percutaneous injection of acrylic bone cement. Radiology 197:307–310

22. Cotten A, Demondion X, Boutry N et al (1999) Therapeutic percutaneous injections in the treatment of malignant acetabular osteolyses. Radiographics 19:647–653

23. Ripamonti C, Twycross R, Baines M et al (2001) Clinical practice recommendations for the management of MBO in patients with end-stage cancer. Support Care Cancer 9:223–233

24. Viola R, Kiteley C and the Supportive Care Guidelines Group (2006) The management of dyspnea in cancer patients: a clinical practice guideline. A quality initiative of the program in evidence-based care (PEBC). Cancer Care Ontario (CCO) Report Date: November 6

25. Jennings AL, Davies AN, Higgins JPT et al (2002) A systematic review of the use of opioids in the management of dyspnea. Thorax 57:939–944

26. Pereira J, Mancini I, Bruera E (2000) The management of bleeding in patients with advanced cancer. In: Portenoy RK, Bruera E (eds) Topics in palliative care, vol. 4. Oxford University Press, New York, pp 163–183

Ethical Aspects in Surgical Oncology

14

P. Celoria

*It is radically wrong to think
we can indicate intelligence as the basic difference
between man and animal: the difference exists on the anatomic
plane, the motor-sensory and that of physiology of the senses.*
A. Gehlen, Man (1940)

A student of Max Scheler and Nicolai Hartmann, Arnold Gehlen was a German anthropologist and philosopher of the twentieth century. His main work "Man, his nature and place in the world" is full of ideas on which to reflect [1].

He was the founder of the philosophical anthropology which opened up the possibility of a series of thoughts on the man-technics relationship, enabling evaluations of an ethical nature in each medical field, in an age that could be defined highly technological.

Gehlen's thought emphasizes it is incorrect to maintain that man possesses "intelligence" more than animals. In actual fact man is lacking in something that animals have: "instinct".

Man does not possess his own environment and does not have physiological capacities that will allow him to survive in each specific condition. But he is a being "open to the world".

This is connected to the fact that he possesses technics – a necessary, unavoidable condition for his very life and essence. Technics is indispensable for him and represents his "second nature".

The myth of Prometheus strengthens the idea of mankind being freed from the animal condition and of complete submission to the gods. The Titan rebels against Zeus and offers men fire, technics. It is through technics that freedom from the yoke of submission comes about. It causes eternal punishment for Prometheus, chained to the Caucasian rock and subjected to the wounds inflicted by the eagle that devoured his liver which continuously grew back again. Aeschylus' "Prometheus Bound" is considered by Galimberti, perhaps rightly, the initial cornerstone of philosophy, understood as the doctrine of the essence and of knowledge.

Language is the first form of technics, enabling man to be free from the need of an immediate driving response and it "exonerates" him from instinctive behaviour

P. Celoria (✉)
Surgical Oncology Unit, S. Giovanni Battista University Hospital, Turin, Italy

New Technologies in Surgical Oncology. Antonio Mussa (Ed.)
© Springer-Verlag Italia 2010

14

[2]. It could be considered as compensation given to man for the fact that he does not possess instinct. By and through technics, therefore, man can survive, evolve and live by projecting himself into the future, in an eternal quest for balance in life and relations.

The surgeon carries out a large part of his healing work profoundly immersed in an intensely technical sphere. The approach to the evaluation, analysis and possible solution of the problems of patients undergoing surgery have always been strongly permeated by technical transductions. It is normal for every surgeon, and for the oncological surgeon, to "act", as Gehlen would observe, with personal psychological and practical responses of an absolutely technical nature in his relationship with the sick person and the disease.

Technical competence itself is ethics for the surgeon. Through technicity he is bent on seeking good in his relations with those requesting assistance and a solution or relief for their suffering. Continuous honing and attentive evaluation of every technical development are part of the legitimate yearning for benevolence, and non-malevolence, in principle, as the basis of moral and deontological behavior.

Our era has witnessed, however, a staggering technical evolution that has brought us to land in an age definable as technological. The condition of reality therefore proceeds, changing continuously. Technics and technology are self-referential. We daily witness events in which it proves clear that from being a means given to man in constituting his second nature, technology has become an end in itself: the aim.

We live in an age in which it is not difficult to come up against a common feeling that says "we should do all we can do", that is, all that technics allow us to do. Therefore, orientation and strategies end up being strongly influenced by technicity and its power; behaviors, ideas, desires and happiness itself seem to belong mainly to the technological conquest and are stimulated and directed by it.

General principles have to stay anchored fast to ethics and politics, meant in the sense Plato indicates in "The Republic", namely the ethics of the *polis* [3]. In the oncological surgeon's work the constant, critical moving towards ethics in the sense of a philosophical doctrine that permeates the life of man and places relational boundaries is as fundamental as knowing in a detailed manner the surgical act and operating procedure.

It is vital to retrieve classical knowledge [3], to resort to one's own sensitivity and human nature in the field of moral philosophy. We need to recall that the surgeon is an intellectual, called to treat and cure people suffering from diseases that are sometimes challenging, like in the oncological sphere. These require technical competence, as well as the capacity for ethical analysis of the overall clinical situation of those who place their trust in the surgeon.

We need to do everything that "should be done and not everything that can be done". Action needs to be controlled with intellectual weapons, since it may constitute the method not conditioned by requests or will dictated by technicity for its own sake. Beside the evidence, then, we also have to draw from the philosophical teachings of our own history that enable us to work better on our own self, so as to offer listening, understanding and the chance to decide for ourselves and for those with expectations for care and healing. Each technical decision will increase in efficacy.

Prometheus is once again topical: the freedom offered to men by fire bound him to despair and suffering. Every oncological surgeon has to undo the chains and go back at this difficult historic moment to evaluating technics and technologies as fundamental and inevitable means and never as the aim of the action carried out. Moral philosophy and the history of Western thought are a valid frame of reference.

The explosion of technology in our era has determined the success of a new, unknown relational modality. The analysis of our own 'I' immersed in a thick, foggy sea of data cannot disregard our own personal call for the moral principles that should accompany all behavior.

The surgeon lives in a condition characterized by impacts and stimuli that are insistent and seductive in terms of technical evolution and healing perspectives. The sick person lives in an identical atmosphere, targeted to the same extent by the same whirlwind of data and proposals, with an interpretation spoilt by reactive anxiety and anguish, as well as by cultural inadequacy. Communicative channels are modulated on the grounds of the interlocutor, never constituting direct or indirect barriers to understanding.

The oncological sphere is psychologically weighted by the type of disease treated, and burdened further by doubts and uncertainties which in the technological era are not understood and endured with difficulty. The cancer patient/oncological surgeon relationship cannot be without reciprocal respect, so as to be safely anchored to a profoundly moral behavioral frame. It is anything but a simple undertaking to define what respect is. In every activity it is not possible to imagine a relationship devoid of respect. In the opposite case, the possibility of reactions not aimed at the common good, far from happiness, is in each individual's feelings.

It is therefore unimaginable that the relationship between the cancer patient and the surgeon not have as its supporting beam, as the very skeleton of the relationship, a pact founded on and impregnated with respect. Nothing efficient, nothing efficacious can materialize if the presuppositions are not founded on this pact, from which originate reciprocal faith, understanding and responsibility.

A particularly crystalline, pure and transparent definition is that proposed by Francisco Torralba, a young Spanish philosopher who recognizes respect as being at an "equidistance between intrusion and indifference" [4]. Analyzing this definition, the concept of equidistance is striking. At each moment in the relationship distance may need to be corrected, and in order to stay so and remain effective, it is in a continuous, incessant state of becoming. It is a subtle art, the commitment for which may sometimes prove enormous. With sick people, with their family members and their expectations, the surgeon and the oncologist have to make considerable efforts to follow and foresee movements of the mind and heart, with the continuous need of the collimation of sensations, to ensure this equidistance. This should translate into an equilibrium that never gives rise to a perception of indifference; but it is just as important that the technical decisions and caring tasks do not translate into intrusion.

Each individual's freedom is sacred, all the more so in sickness. Disinterested, correct information and education are the tools for the dialogue with those seeking care and treatment, with the aim of allowing perception of the respect that must involve the person in his totality, human, social and affective. This should occur both in the acute phase of the disease, and as it continues, both for the operation and in the periods following the operation.

Respect cannot be but reciprocal. It is not possible to imagine surgery carried out on a person not offering the surgeon respect both for his person and the technique proposed and implemented. This is obtained through active, meaningful communicative work, devoid of fear, sincere and aimed at the common good. Management of the relational balance can only initially be on the part of the surgeon or doctor, who far from any paternalistic attitude is intellectually and technically organised to offer and obtain that equidistance which translates into a balance of reciprocal understanding, a constantly evolving communicative act. He who seeks care, and whose autonomy and inviolability are respectfully acknowledged, frequently becomes a "teacher" to those offering assistance.

In a society where often those who shout the loudest are the strongest, where communication is spoilt by non-neutral technology, where expectations become a source of anxiety and suffering, the theme of listening is of primary importance. Doctors are quite often accused of not listening. They are charged with indifference and protagonism, indeed for "not listening".

Listening is an art. For the oncological surgeon it is an absolute necessity. From the technical point of view listening to each of the patient's tales, guided, too, by maieutics, perfects moments of diagnosis, enabling the relationship to begin well. Listening is an intentional act, a wilful act. It has the objective of understanding the other. It is a free act whose antechamber is silence.

Every doctor knows that he has to face his patient's problems with a clear mind, putting himself into the relationship with an attitude of true listening that must be perceived by the person suffering. By being silent he enters into contact, preparing the relationship for listening and being listened to. Silence is seen as the antechamber of listening.

Francisco Torralba, once again, in the chapter of his book devoted to sick people, "The art of listening", puts forward an ethical theme on which to reflect. He maintains that "there are circumstances in which the only worthy attitude is seriousness. Seriousness is an ethical requirement, connected with responsibility, constancy and commitment, without deception or meanness. This does not prevent us from laughing at our own seriousness. Sick people can speak authoritatively of the dark side of life, of the fragility of our condition, powerlessness in the face of harm and suffering" [4].

To train oneself to be silent, to listen and be listened to is an ethical requirement for the oncological surgeon. From good listening the relationship is placed on a track aimed at bearing fruit.

Medical culture is based ethically on listening and action in terms of the sick person, listening and action which are free from any prejudice or critical attitude for its own sake. The purpose is always and only that of recognizing evidence and lawfulness of the medical act, with the aims of achieving the result intended.

Intellectual understanding means analysis independent of emotional facts. The boundary of participation becomes subtle, sometimes imperceptible, rich in behavioral pitfalls. In their actions surgeons have on the one hand the ethical and technical need to relate with their patients, and on the other, the awareness that unguided emotional involvement produces damage for oneself and for the person being helped, with a loss in efficacy.

Through the concept of equidistance between intrusion and indifference, continuously being modified in the relationship, the reference frame for his own action needs to be found.

The ethical approach for the surgeon, therefore, has three fundamental criteria: firstly, to break down any emotional participation during the operation, secondly, to develop technicity to obtain results aimed at good, and thirdly, to show empathy, the effort to link intellectually, with no moral judgements or affective involvement, aimed at understanding the other and his requests. As Vladimir Jankélévitch, a moral philosopher for thirty years at the Sorbonne, states, "it is not a question of being virtuous: one just needs to be serious and faithful" [5].

Deontologically, a sense of responsibility should be borne in mind which does not admit any delegation. Remember that some twenty per cent of communication is verbal, and that language, postural and mimetic, should not be underestimated in the slightest. Bear in mind that listening as availability, suited to time, place and manner, is an art that cannot be refrained from, and that respect, equidistance between intrusion and indifference, will sooner or later be perceived by the other and evaluated. One needs to concentrate on governing one's own and the other's technological conditioning.

In recent years an increasingly evident phenomenon has been witnessed, characterized by a medical and surgical attitude based on defence. Defence of one's own work, with respect to the continually rising number of cases brought against healthcare operators for the purpose of compensation and proceedings of a penal nature. The defensive attitude is in clear contrast with the ethical principles that animate surgery work, although it is humanly understandable and sometimes unavoidable.

Each procedure, be it in the diagnostic or therapeutic sphere, cannot be but totally aligned with the concept of lawfulness and necessity, once the alternatives have been technically evaluated. It is obvious that reasoning which breaks away from this concept based on the ethical principle places the surgeon in a condition of suffering and alienation. Making decisions about a patient, whatever they may be, for reasons not strictly correlated with good and respect for clinical dictates cannot even be considered.

The challenge of retrieving the role, the ethical struggle with what conditions the relationship with the patient, of transforming action into something to demonstrate to third parties and not to suffer personal consequences is great. The reference to philosophy and thought, free from conditioning, may, at least partly, enable that retrieval.

In this sense medical work and surgery cannot disregard teaching. Teaching is an essential, basic moment of acting. In each decision, each act of diagnosis or treatment, the aspect of sharing with a colleague and educating those who are not experts is intrinsic. Teaching and training are integral parts of ethics. According to Greek thought, integrity and unity should always be considered as almost indissoluble from the two moments, ethics and didactics, within a single intent.

Oncological surgeons need to feel convinced of the need to pass on their own experience to younger people. They should share with them their own doubts, in a critical sense, pointing out the complexity of their actions. They should listen to objections and requests with a free spirit, so as to be able to offer concrete answers to often crucial questions. They should constantly refer back to ethical-deontological principles in teaching, in order to draw the attention of those learning to the proper behavioral modalities, to obtain solid training.

A difficult moment in teaching is to offer the tools for rendering the theoretical knowledge acquired operative. University training is particularly rich in information and constitutes an inalienable theoretical base. The translation of this wealth of knowledge into practical application shows intrinsic difficulty, which should be evaluated and tackled.

We need to make the effort to have it understood how absolutely important the times are that schooling devotes to bringing the student close to the patient, during which teaching should concern, together with and as worthy as, technical aspects, ethical and deontological issues.

Oncological disease is manifold. Oncological surgeons are faced each day with people who rightly await answers and solutions. They must be free and serene in their actions, convinced of the potential of technicity and of the need to use it as a means aimed at the good of their patients and their own, to further enhance synergism.

Aeschylus' tragedy "Prometheus Bound" is paradigmatic. Technology, apparatuses, media, personalisms are invisible chains which hamper action, making it defensive and impersonal, sometimes far from the true end, which is still nevertheless happiness, even in such situations of disease as conflictual as those of oncology. Moral philosophy and the retrieval of the tradition of Western thought can help to break these chains.

The oncological surgeon is a technician who cannot forget also being an intellectual, capable of listening, able to avoid conditioning while taking responsibility for decisions and offering the equidistance between indifference and intrusion on which respect is founded.

Hippocrates, whose oath is sworn by every oncological surgeon, invites every doctor to be a philosopher. Ethics is didactics, and every doctor knows that it is ethical to teach and train younger people, whereas neglecting this role is unethical.

Enabling the legacy to be alive and be continually renewed and enriched is a moral commitment. In preparing young doctors the absolute valorization of training periods is obligatory, during which they should be guided in approaching the patient. The objective is twofold: confirmation of theoretical knowledge and reflection on philosophical aspects. The university might feel the need to institute a moral philosophy course during the early years of the degree course, together with, and as noble as, technical subjects, as well as enhancing the study of the history of medicine.

A page by Louis-Ferdinand Céline taken from "Mort à crédit", published in 1936, deserves some comments [6]. Céline is one of the most controversial personalities of twentieth century literature. Harshly criticized for his anti-Semitism, he practised his profession after the First World War as a general practitioner in popular districts of Paris. In the story he confides in his cousin Gustin Sabayot, a few years older than himself, also a doctor and an expert. He goes home with the latter after a hard day's work and, awaiting dinner, tells him of his tiredness. Gustin answers him, suffering from cynicism and pessimism that are truly worrying:

"Do you think they're ill? ... One moans ... another belches ... that one staggers ... this one is covered in boils ... Do you want to empty the waiting-room? Instantly? ... even of those who keep on spitting till their chest will burst? Suggest a bash of cinema! ... a free aperitif, thrown in their face! ... you'll see how many will stay ... If they come looking for you, it's mostly because they're bored. There's not a chance you'll see one on the eve of a feast-day ... The wretches need a job, not health, remember what I tell you ... They simply need you to distract them, put them in a good mood, be interested in their burps ... their gas ... their creaking ... discover their wind ... their little fevers ... their rumbling ... what a novelty! Take time over them ... get interested ... that's why you've got your degree ... Ah! Enjoy yourself with your own death while you're creating it, that's all Man is, Ferdinand! Let that lot keep their dribbling, their syphilis, their tubercles. They need them! And their bladders full of slime and their backsides on fire, they couldn't care less about all that! But if you get busy, if you're able to interest them, they will wait for you to die, it's your reward! They'll come and dig you out till the end."

It is best to bear in mind for oneself and one's own students that this sentiment may be hidden in each person. Know it. Control it. So that it does no harm.

References

1. Gehlen A (1988) Man: his nature and place in the world. Columbia University Press, New York
2. Galimberti U (1999) Psiche e techne. L'uomo nell'età della tecnica (Psyche and technics. Man in the age of technicity). Feltrinelli, Milan
3. Russell B (1945) A history of Western philosophy. Simon and Schuster, New York.
4. Torralba F (2006) L'arte di ascoltare ("The art of listening"). Rizzoli, Milan
5. Jankélévitch V (1962) Corso di filosofia morale. Raffaello Cortina Editore, Milan
6. Céline L-F (1936) Mort à crédit. Garzanti, Milan

Suggested Readings

Heidegger M (1929) What is metaphysics? Adelphi, Milan
Galimberti U (2000) Idee: il catalogo è questo ("Ideas: the catalogue is this"), Feltrinelli, Milan
Galimberti U (2007) L'ospite inquietante (The worrying guest) Rizzoli, Milan
Review 'Hermeneutica' (2007) Corpo e persona (Body and person), Morcelliana, Brescia

Subject Index

Printed in October 2009